An Ounce of Prevention

MIT Press Series in Health and Public Policy
Jeffrey E. Harris, general editor

1. *Professionalism and the Public Interest: Price and Quality in Optometry*, James W. Begun, 1981.

2. *Controlling Hospital Costs: The Role of Government Regulation*, Paul L. Joskow, 1981.

3. *Biomedical Innovation*, edited by Edward B. Roberts, Robert I. Levy, Stan N. Finkelstein, Jay Moskowitz, and Edward J. Sondik, 1981.

4. *An Ounce of Prevention: Child Health Politics under Medicaid*, Anne-Marie Foltz, 1982.

An Ounce of Prevention

Child Health Politics under Medicaid

Anne-Marie Foltz

The MIT Press
Cambridge, Massachusetts, and London, England

This book was set in Palatino by Graphic Composition, Inc., and printed and bound in the United States of America.

Library of Congress Cataloging in Publication Data

Foltz, Anne-Marie.
  An ounce of prevention.

(MIT Press series in health and public policy   ; 4)

  Bibliography: p.
  Includes index.
  1. Early and Periodic Screening, Diagnosis, and Treatment Program. 2. Child health services—Government policy—United States. I. Title. II. Series. [DNLM: 1. Child health services—United States. 2. Child welfare—United States. 3. Health policy—United States. 4. Medical assistance, Title 19. W1 MI938 v. 4 / WA 320 F6710]
RJ102.F55   362.1'9892'000973   81–23655
ISBN 0–262–06082–5   AACR2

To Bill

As princes do in times of action get
New taxes, and remit them not in peace,
No winter shall abate this spring's increase.

John Donne

Contents

Series Foreword   xi
Preface   xiii
Tables   xv
Abbreviations   xvii

Introduction: The Politics of Prevention   1

I   Formation and Implementation of Child Health Policy under Medicaid   11

1   The Development of EPSDT   13
The First Building Block: Title V   13
The Second Building Block: Medicaid (Title XIX)   16
Legacies of Titles V and XIX   20
Beginnings of EPSDT   22
Regulations and Guidelines   29

2   Implementation   36
Congressional Neglect   36
HEW's Neglect   37
Resolving Ambiguities: The States Have a Try   41
Incrementalism at Work   59

II   Institutional Constraints   61

3   Federal-State Relations   63
Grants and Compliance   64
The EPSDT Penalty   65
Reasons for the Penalty's Failure   67
Limits of Federalism   75

4   Health and Welfare Ideologies   *78*
Welfare Department Goals   *80*
Health Department Goals   *88*
Is Organizational Ideology a Constraint?   *97*

5   Bureaucratic Capacity:
Case Management Systems   *99*
Federal Assistance for State Management   *100*
Connecticut   *101*
Texas   *107*
Is Bureaucratic Capacity a Constraint?   *114*
Institutional Constraints   *115*

III   The Technological Constraint:
Is There a Consensus?   *117*

6   Searching for a Consensus on Standards
for Child Health Care   *119*
Defining Terms   *119*
Origins of the Periodic Health Examination   *121*
Special Risks and Needs of Children   *124*
Search for Consensus on Standards   *129*
What Are the Standards for Preventive Care?   *139*
Is There Consensus?   *153*

7   What do Policy-Makers Know and
When do They Know It?   *155*
The Swine Flu Fiasco   *155*
Making Immunizations Mandatory   *157*
The Frequency of Screening Under EPSDT   *159*
The Technological Constraint   *163*

Conclusion: Politics, Prevention,
and Policy   *167*

Appendix 1
Events Relating to EPSDT Regulations and Enforcement, and to the Proposed CHAP, 1972–1980   181

Appendix 2
Pediatric Textbooks, Reference and Practice Books, and Preventive Medicine Books   185

Appendix 3
Persons Interviewed   192

Notes   195

Bibliography   231

Index   249

Series Foreword

This MIT Press series serves as a forum for significant new research in the field of health and public policy. The series encompasses current problems in health-care organization, financing, and regulation. It also focuses on emerging policy problems in environmental health, workplace safety, toxic substances, and the assessment of new medical technology. We plan to publish original scholarly monographs, highly focused collections by multiple authors, and textbooks that explore new fields.

In this fourth volume in the Health and Public Policy Series, Anne-Marie Foltz of New York University examines the origins and fate of the Early and Periodic Screening, Diagnosis, and Treatment Program of Medicaid. Three main issues emerge from her analysis. First, the success of an innovative public health policy hinges critically on the creation of a scientific consensus on its effectiveness. Second, the structure of federal-state relations in the United States plays a central role in the implementation of national health care initiatives. Third, a strategy of gradual, incremental change, although typical of American democratic institutions, may be inappropriate for many public health policies. Dr. Foltz has made a major contribution to the current debate on the role of government in the provision of preventive health care.

Jeffrey E. Harris

Preface

In 1972 I began studying Medicaid's child health program, EPSDT, and have been writing intermittently about it since. A disadvantage of getting to know one's subject too well is that it becomes like an old friend: one is reluctant to reveal its weaknesses lest one be responsible for rendering it vulnerable. What we study begins to become a part of our lives. We begin to have an affection for it, and it gets more difficult to maintain scholarly detachment. This may extend not only to the policy itself, but to the persons who work with it. For information and understanding, I have been dependent on these people. They have been cooperative, friendly, and informative. In respecting their dedication to their work, I have found it difficult to discuss the program lest some comment allow abuse to be heaped on it.

Medicaid, with its long history of purported abuse and fraud, and EPSDT, with its long history of inaction, have generated large numbers of well-meaning harpies ready to attack at the program's first sign of weakness. Moreover, although it is popular and acceptable in the press to blame the bureaucrats and the recipients of services for misusing funds, the providers of such services (except for nursing homes) have remained relatively immune from attack. This study also will focus mainly on the bureaucrats, and only indirectly on the providers and recipients.

Thus, this study of constraints on the implementation of Medicaid/EPSDT policy for children may aid, abet, and comfort those who would advocate its demise, because the program fails to do properly what some thought it was supposed to do regardless of measurable or unmeasurable, tangible or intangible benefits. Nevertheless, I hope that my analysis of this federal policy can provide lessons on how to implement state and federal policy, and that it will not serve as a prescription for eliminating health care for poor children—a case of throwing out the baby with the bath water.

I am grateful to many friends who have helped me in this study. George A. Silver, by inviting me to join the Yale Health Policy Project, and by sharing his vast knowledge, first launched me on the study of child health. Stephen S. Mick patiently and warmly supervised this study in its original form as a Yale dissertation. Rose-mary A. Stevens, by her encouragement and by the example of her work, inspired this "Son of Medicaid." James W. Fesler introduced me to the intricacies of public administration and the appreciation of clear writing.

The state and federal officials, scholars, and child health advocates interviewed for this study were gracious with their time and information. They are listed in appendix 3. This study could not have been written without their generous help. I am particularly grateful to Beatrice Moore, Chapin Wilson, Estelle Siker, and Bob Smith for repeated conversations.

The National Center for Health Services Research, Department of Health, Education, and Welfare, made this study possible by providing Dissertation Grant HS–02852 from 1977 to 1979. The grant also permitted me to work with two able research assistants, Carol De Canio and Judith Blamey.

Special thanks go to John Butler, George D. Greenberg, Wendy Lazarus, Helen Martz, C. Arden Miller, Beatrice Moore, and two anonymous reviewers for MIT Press who provided copious cogent comment on entire drafts of this manuscript. My appreciation also to those who provided suggestions for portions of the work in progress at various times: David Abrahamsen, Marlin Johnston, Stephen Press, Dennis Smith, and Helen D. Ward.

I owe thanks to my colleagues on the New Haven Board of Aldermen and my many political friends and opponents in New Haven, who from 1973 to 1978 showed me how implementation politics really works.

Beverly Cedarbaum brilliantly negotiated my inconsistencies, my handwriting, and my chaotic typing to produce the penultimate and ultimate drafts of this manuscript. Martha Achilles assisted with the bibliography.

These acknowledgments would not be complete without noting the considerable contribution of the Foltz household. Peter W. Foltz and Jeremy D. Foltz calculated percentages, searched references, xeroxed, proof-read, and goaded me on by threatening to graduate before I did. William J. Foltz's services as chief counsel, editor, and tea-bearer reflect only a small part of his contribution. He made completion of this study plausible, and ultimately possible.

All my friends and relatives have provided much advice—most of it good. If I have failed to benefit, they are not responsible.

Tables

1 Federal expenditures and services for children under twenty-one provided by Title V and Title XIX (Medicaid) of the Social Security Act (selected years) *Page* 17

2 Children eligible for and screened by the EPSDT program, by state, 1973, 1976, 1978 49

3 EPSDT and Medicaid services in selected states 52

4 States mandating immunizations prior to school entry 141

5 Primary immunizations recommended by the American Academy of Pediatrics, Report of the Committee on Infectious Diseases ("Red Book") 144

6 Average number of recommended physician visits for each age group: Pediatric and preventive medicine text and reference books 150

7 Number of recommended screening visits for each age group: Academy of Pediatrics 150

8 Recommended number of screening visits by age group: Assorted individuals and organizations, 1973–1977 152

9 Number of screenings paid for by state EPSDT programs by age, 1977 160

Appendix 1 Events Relating to EPSDT Penalty Regulations and Enforcement and to the Proposed CHAP, 1972–1980. 181

Appendix 2 Pediatric Textbooks, Reference and Practice Books, and Preventive Medicine Books 185

Abbreviations

AAP	American Academy of Pediatrics
AB	Aid to the Blind
AFDC	Aid to Families with Dependent Children
APTD	Aid to the Permanently and Totally Disabled
CC	Crippled Children's (Program)
CDF	Children's Defense Fund
CETA	Comprehensive Employment Training Act
CHAP	Child Health Assurance Program (earlier known as Child Health Assessment Program)
C&Y	Children and Youth (Project)
EMIC	Emergency Maternity and Infant Care (Program)
FSII	Field Staff Information and Instruction Series
HCFA	Health Care Financing Administration
HEW	U.S. Department of Health, Education, and Welfare
HHS	U.S. Department of Health and Human Services
HMO	Health Maintenance Organization
JCQA	Joint Committee on Quality Assurance
MCH	Maternal and Child Health (Program)
MCHS	Maternal and Child Health Services
MIC	Maternity and Infant Care (Project)
MMIS	Medical Management Information System
MSA	Medical Services Administration
NCSS	National Center for Social Statistics
OCH	Office of Child Health
OMB	U.S. Office of Management and Budget
SRS	Social and Rehabilitation Service
SSI	Supplementary Security Income

Introduction: The Politics of Prevention

We look toward the day when every child, no matter what his color or his family's means, gets the medical care he needs.
Lyndon B. Johnson
8 February 1967

This is a study of the Early and Periodic Screening, Diagnosis, and Treatment Program (EPSDT) of Medicaid (Title XIX). It is about a federal program signed into law in 1968 with the intention of providing preventive and curative health services for poor children. It is about a federal program which failed to reach its potential of providing preventive care to 12 percent of America's children, but nevertheless managed to provide for millions of them who would otherwise never have received it.

The program was born in 1966 out of a Department of Health, Education, and Welfare (HEW) program analysis and signed into law by President Johnson on 2 January 1968. As an amendment to Title XIX of the Social Security Act, which had been enacted in 1965 and provided payments for medical services for the poor, EPSDT required that the states provide for

such early and periodic screening and diagnosis of individuals who are eligible under the plan and are under the age of 21 to ascertain their physical or mental defects and such health care, treatment, and other measures to correct or ameliorate defects and chronic conditions discovered thereby, as may be provided in regulations of the Secretary.[1]

Although the Title XIX program had previously provided payment for treatment, this was the first time that the states were required to provide preventive health and screening services with the requisite follow-up treatment as needed. At the time, approximately ten million children were eligible for such Medicaid services, which made this potentially the most significant and far-reaching child health program the federal government had ever undertaken.

The EPSDT amendments had slipped through Congress late in 1967 with little comment. Final regulations did not emerge from HEW until November 1971 with full implementation not required until mid-1973. Under the regulations, the states were required to provide for screening for all eligible children as well as necessary follow-up treatment, including dental, vision, and hearing care, even though the states had not previously provided such services.

States responded to the requirements almost as slowly as HEW had responded to the requirement of drafting regulations. They had to seek out those children eligible, find providers of services, draw up periodicity schedules for screening, set standards, and, theoretically, monitor the program. If all this seemed a bit much for the states, they were the first to say so.

The program had some limited success. Each year the number of children reached by the program increased. In 1978, over two million children were screened through the program, and an unknown number of these children treated for ailments found. The costs of the program remained relatively modest as federal social programs go. Even as late as 1976, annual screening costs alone were only $47 million, or less than 0.3 percent of all Medicaid expenditures.[2] Moreover, the costs for diagnosis and treatment of the children had not risen in most states in greater proportions than the costs of Medicaid services to the adult population, which lacked such a screening program.

Nevertheless, by 1975 HEW and state implementation of the program had been roundly condemned by the Congress which had enacted it.[3] A House Subcommittee accused HEW of "mismanagement" in implementing the program.[4] Others, outside Congress, decried the program as "abominable," a public waste of unnecessary screening,[5] or simply a failure.[6] Even EPSDT's most ardent advocates acknowledged that its record had "not been impressive."[7] Within less than ten years of its inception, Congress began several unsuccessful attempts to improve the program. The failure of these legislative revisions ultimately left the program in the 1980s as an unhappy stepchild having difficulty proving its worth to a skeptical and conservative executive branch.

The objective of this study is to determine why this ambitious program of services, mandated by federal law, was so poorly implemented. The EPSDT program was the first federal attempt to purchase directly preventive and curative ambulatory care services for poor children and to require state agencies to manage that care. The problems this program encountered in its first ten years indicate the problems any third party might encounter in buying ambulatory care services for a population when these services are not readily available. They indicate as well the problems state agencies have in managing continuity between preventive and follow-up care. This case history of EPSDT/Medicaid illustrates the constraints under which any publicly financed health services program must operate.

Health programs may be classified as closed or open systems. In a closed system, once a patient or client is enrolled in a program or clinic, he has little choice beyond that group of who provides his health services. Health Maintenance Organizations (HMOs) are typical of closed systems. Neighborhood health centers and most other publicly financed clinics are also closed systems in that they are established to serve geographically and often categorically designated clientele.

In contrast, an open system such as EPSDT/Medicaid permits the client to choose among a wide range of providers of health services. For example, in theory, a Medicaid-eligible child has the right to go to any pediatrician or general practitioner or health clinic for services. The "right" is theoretical because health providers may refuse—and many do refuse—to see Medicaid patients, but this does not change the basic structure of the system.

Closed systems may have some disadvantages for the client in that they offer little choice of provider. However, what they lose in provider flexibility they make up for in administrative simplicity. Under such closed systems, data are stored in one place and all providers are employed under the same administrative auspices; therefore billing, payment, and oversight are simplified. Open systems where providers work independently of one another are administratively cumbersome.

Most health services in the United States are delivered through the open system. In 1978, only 3 percent of the U.S. population was served by HMOs. Meanwhile, the Medicaid program alone served three times that number.[8]

EPSDT, as an open system to provide both preventive and treatment services for children, approximates the present system of health care available for most persons in the United States; therefore, the EPSDT experience can be considered a significant natural experiment in health administration whose results should have implications for new programs which seek marginal, rather than structural, reforms of the present health care system.

The judgment that the EPSDT program has failed is similar to that which commentators passed on many of the social service programs instituted during the Great Society's leap forward in the 1960s. These programs have been studied by a host of political scientists, sociologists, economists, and lawyers.[9] This study seeks to build on their work, keeping in mind that failure is defined by the goals of a program. If the goals are unclear, as they turned out to be in the case of the EPSDT program, assessment of "success" or "failure" becomes a futile pursuit. This study, then, is in the tradition of implementation studies, not evaluations.[10]

All programs are implemented by institutions. Within these institutions individuals or groups of individuals make decisions as to what actions should be taken. For most social service programs these institutions are already in place when a federal law or policy is enacted. For Medicaid and the EPSDT program these institutions were the Department of Health, Education, and Welfare at the federal level, and state health and welfare agencies. Each of these institutions had its own goals, traditions, objectives, internal politics, and capacities. An institution when confronted by a new program may try earnestly to carry it out and may succeed in doing so; or it may carry out the program only partially because it lacks the capacity or because other programs take precedence and draw off scarce institutional resources; it may also simply refuse to carry out a program because it conflicts with its own goals or operational traditions, or because it may require coordination with or subordination to rival agencies. Such institutional factors may constrain implementation of a program which on paper looked reasonable and useful.[11]

Two intellectual traditions are useful in attempting to explain why institutions in our political system succeed or fail in carrying out programs. The first tradition is that on decision-making. In thinking about social programs, we tend to assume that legislators and bureaucrats are rational actors who shape programs to their own ends. In fact, as scholars have increasingly shown, this is not the way decisions are reached.

Administrators make their decisions not necessarily on the basis of an overall grand plan or strategy but by a series of incremental steps where means and ends are not clearly distinguished. This incremental problem-solving technique permits administrators to function under the usual constraints of real world decision-making; when information is insufficient, when they are under conflicting pressures, when theoretical underpinnings for policy are unavailable, or when no action is worse than some action.[12] Decisions are often made through mutual adjustment, in which competing agencies or individuals slowly modify their preferences so as to establish a compromise outcome which each side can tolerate.

The functioning of such a system is illustrated in Allison's study of decision-making in the Cuban missile crisis in which he showed that the best explanation for the decisions made came not from using a rational actor model, but a "bureaucratic politics" model based on the assumption that bureaucracies are not monolithic and that they permit disagreement among reasonable men about what is to be done.[13] Similar patterns of adjustment also occur in Congress where a congressman's voting behavior can be explained by the system of rewards and incentives available to him within the Congress and within his electorate.[14]

Under the American system of values, this incremental decision-making process is considered to be worthwhile regardless of the programs and policies which may result from the decisions. Thus one need not be entirely discouraged that programs do not always achieve their goals, because the political process is valuable in and of itself. As Lindblom argues, the public interest is achieved by individuals going through this process of mutual adjustment in order to move toward values they believe shared.[15] One need not agree with Lindblom's normative judgments about the desirability of such behavior in order to accept the findings that institutions do in fact function that way and that the modes of analysis employed to study them yield powerful empirical explanations of outcomes.

In true "incremental" fashion, EPSDT's policy goals were not clearly stated at the outset. In part I, I shall present EPSDT's legislative origins in the earlier federal child health policies of the Title V (Maternal and Child Health) programs and the Medicaid program. I shall then present EPSDT's ambiguous legislative development, its administrative neglect by HEW, and its slow and imperfect implementation by the states during its first decade.

The second intellectual tradition which helps explain program success and failure stems from "implementation studies," that is, studies of how institutions actually order programs into being and carry them out. Four of these studies represent the best in this tradition and suggest explanations for program failure and success. Three studies are of federal social programs and all involve failures of one degree or another. They are Title V of the Elemen-

tary and Secondary Education Act (ESEA),[16] economic development in Oakland, California,[17] and "new towns in-town."[18] The
fourth of these is about the Polaris missile development program,
which was a success, perhaps because it had a technological rather
than a social goal.[19]

Federal inability to get localities to carry out federal goals was an
institutional constraint noted for the new towns program. The
complexity of federal-local relationships demonstrated the limits
of centralization in our political system. This limited federal influence also appeared in the Oakland unemployment and the ESEA
educational studies. Unlike new towns and the unemployment
program, the EPSDT program required state agencies, not the localities, to carry out the program. Whether federal control could
have any more success dealing with state bureaucracies and
whether this weakness inherent in federal power was an important factor in explaining the poor implementation of EPSDT is a
question which is explored in the beginning of part II.

A second institutional constraint develops from the distinct cultures of organizations manifest in their ideologies and statements
of goals. As Murphy noted, "This organizational culture is manifest in a history, traditions, norms, accepted ways of conducting
business, and standard operating procedures."[20] Murphy's study
looked at the same organizations operating within different state
contexts. In the case of EPSDT, not only were there fifty different
states, but in many states there were at least two agencies, health
and welfare, each with its own traditions and each given or desir-
ing partial responsibility for, or control over, the program. Different organizational cultures and ideologies, and different
interpretations of proper instrumental goals therefore become another set of institutional constraints within which the EPSDT program had to operate.

A third institutional constraint stems from the issues of bureaucratic capacity to deal with programs. The ability to manage technological complexity was considered one of three prime factors for
the success of the Polaris missile program. The EPSDT program,
which combined a technological health program with a social program, thereby required great management capacity. The ability of
state agencies to cope with EPSDT's requirements is also explored
as a major constraint on the program.

These are then the three institutional constraints to implementation of the EPSDT program which are discussed in part II. Each

of the constraints is analyzed for its effect on EPSDT and also for whether the constraint can be overcome in such a setting.

Agreement on values may also be critical for the success of a program. In the Polaris missile study, the fact that there was a consensus on national needs which could be met by the program, and that there was an available technological solution were significant factors in the program's success.[21] This consensus is so rare, Sapolsky believes, that the only examples prior to Polaris were the Manhattan and Apollo projects.[22] Such consensus may be even more difficult to achieve in social service programs, which may explain the limits of applying technological solutions to social problems.[23] The technological solutions proposed for social programs may be, at best, untried and, at worst, totally unsuitable.

EPSDT, as a health program and like the Polaris missile program, incorporated the use of a technology. The scientific values of a screening program were incorporated into EPSDT's legal basis, although screening was, in fact, an untried technology. Nevertheless, this technology of screening was highly valued in the medical community during the mid-1960s. As it turned out, the technology of screening and preventive care came increasingly under fire as being inappropriate, and no consensus on national need was ever established. Therefore, the program may well have lacked the consensus which, at least in other studies, has been judged as critical to success. The road to successful implementation is so hazardous that such consensus may be necessary to keep the various administrative agencies at work rather than at each other's throats. How this consensus of the 1960s on screening evaporated without being replaced by any other consensus on national need nor any other clear technology is the subject of "the technological constraint" discussed in part III.

Having taken the reader this far, I need to explain two key words in this study's title, "prevention" and "politics." Prevention in its most general sense means to keep an anticipated event from occurring. In the phrase "preventive medicine," the word has been in use since at least the seventeenth century to mean a substance taken to ward off disease, a prophylactic.[24]

In the twentieth century the term has taken on additional meanings. Preventive medicine is the study and application of all types of prevention, by warding off the anticipated event not only through medicine but also through other means. Clinicians have dropped the distinction between prevention and preventive medicine and merged them into a single concept of prevention. Primary prevention is considered the actual prevention of disease whether it is through the application of a particular measure such as an immunization against poliomyelitis, or whether it involves health education, or the removal of a carcinogenic agent from a person's environment. Secondary prevention is the early detection of disease, usually through screening, when it is believed that the progress of the disease can be arrested through appropriate intervention.[25]

The EPSDT program, as we shall see in parts I and III, was born out of these perceptions of prevention, and the screening program was viewed as an important way of preventing disease among needy children. That the efficacy of screening had never seriously been tested in any but a few programs was not fully realized at the time. At any rate, the EPSDT program was an attempt to make primary and secondary preventive health services available to the most needy children in America.

Politics, according to an established definition, is the issue of who gets what, when, and how.[26] This usually means the way in which exchanges of power take place within a social system and the way costs and benefits are allocated among different groups of people. This understanding of politics is ordinarily applied to a political system, political parties, voting behavior of the public, the actions of elected representatives, and the distribution of public goods and services. However, politics also operates within and between all institutions; and I mean politics in this broader sense. A program is shaped by the politics of all the institutions or agencies through which it passes and these institutional decisions are in turn shaped by needs, rivalries, and power plays. Implementation politics may be a particularly virulent and defensive form of politics because, as Bardach noted,

it is a form of politics in which the very existence of an already defined policy mandate, legally and legitimately authorized in some prior political process, affects the strategy and tactics of the struggle. . . . The outcome of such defensive politics of this sort is delay, a dispersion of energies toward highly particularistic program goals, and, often, a flight from administrative or political responsibility.[27]

In this sense, then, the politics of the EPSDT program implementation cannot be divorced from the political origins of the program. This study involves politics up and down the line from EPSDT's birth by vote of Congress to its shaky childhood in the hands of state health and welfare agencies.

Research for this study was carried out through analysis of internal and published agency documents and through extensive interviews with public officials in Washington and in two states, Connecticut and Texas. I chose the former state because I could build on my earlier work on the EPSDT program. I then asked HEW officials to suggest several states they perceived as having successful case management systems which could serve as a contrast with Connecticut. Texas was ultimately picked because it had as well a large number of children eligible for services, and a poor distribution of health providers, particularly in rural areas, which increased the contrast with Connecticut. Interviews with federal and Connecticut officials took place at different times throughout 1977 and 1978. The Texas interviews took place mainly during February 1978 and were followed by telephone conversations to complete data collection. Federal and state officials also provided data on the program's services, as well as public documents and memos.[28]

The study of ideologies of health and welfare departments relies primarily on the systematic analysis of annual reports from those two departments in Connecticut and Texas. Research on the technological constraint, the consensus on pediatric preventive care, was carried out through a systematic review of pediatric textbooks and handbooks, and the publications of the American Academy of Pediatrics from 1930 to the present.[29]

The purpose of this study, then, is twofold. First, it seeks to examine EPSDT as an example of incremental policy-making. Second, it seeks to explain EPSDT's imperfect implementation by examining four possible constraints—three which derive from institutional characteristics and one which derives from the state of scientific medical knowledge. By such an examination of one public program for a selected group of children it becomes possible to consider how such public programs might operate if extended to other populations, and to assess where their strengths and weaknesses lie.

I Formation and Implementation of Child Health Policy under Medicaid

It will be very bad economy if we continue to save money in this country at the cost of the bodies and the minds and the souls of American children.

C. E. A. Winslow (1940)

1   *The Development of EPSDT*

The formation and implementation of the EPSDT program is a good example of incremental decision-making at its best and worst: at its best if one believes that policy-making in a pluralist democracy is best accomplished through small steps and slow stages; at its worst if one focuses on the confusions, ambiguities, and uncertainties which plagued the program and much of child health policy during the 1970s.

The EPSDT program grew out of two federal programs, Titles V and XIX of the Social Security Act, each with its own philosophy, administrative structure, and financing. It was a hybrid child of different political philosophies of public involvement in child health care. To build on both these programs simultaneously, which is what Congress did in enacting the EPSDT amendments in 1967, is to act instrumentally and incrementally. In no way was EPSDT to differ substantially from earlier programs. That these programs might have conflicting goals and philosophies was an issue not raised in EPSDT's formation. Nor did it become a major part of the discussions in 1977–1980, when Congress was considering revisions of the EPSDT program. The resulting policy, particularly in its early years, was ambiguous—uncertain in its financing, administrative structure, clientele, and the types of care it was to provide.

The First Building Block: Title V

The federal government had entered only reluctantly into the business of providing health services to children. The first federal program to provide such care through grants-in-aid to the states, the Sheppard-Towner Act of 1921, established a pattern for federal grants-in-aid to the states.[1] State health departments were to use federal funds to improve their capacity to promote the "welfare and hygiene of maternity and infancy." The language of the law reflected the beginning of a continuing problem in federal policy—the statement of broad goals with little clarification. But it also established governmental interest in programs of prevention. At that time, the promotion of maternal and infant hygiene was considered to be best accomplished through good nutrition, regular medical checks, good sanitation, and general education for mothers. (See part III for the development of these notions of prevention.) These ideas of prevention were translated into services provided for the most part in well-child conferences. The law also established the precedent, not without a struggle, that the program was to be administered from the federal level by the Children's Bureau (at that time lodged in the Department of Labor) and not by the Public Health Service.[2] The Children's Bureau had been formed in 1912 through an act of Congress and had gradually taken on more and more tasks, not only reporting on the state of child welfare as called for in its original mandate, but promoting programs and legislation to improve the lot of children.

The financing for this impressive mandate was relatively modest. Less than a million dollars per year had been spent by the time the program expired in 1929, with three states, Connecticut, Illinois, and Massachusetts, having chosen not to participate on the grounds that the law infringed on states' rights.[3]

Although the Sheppard-Towner Act died in 1929 through the organized efforts of the American Medical Association and through the lack of support from many of its former friends, particularly the women's groups,[4] many of its goals and structures were revived in 1935 with the passage of Title V of the Social Security Act. It maintained the same federal-state relationship of grants-in-aid to state health departments and the same federal administering agency, the Children's Bureau. It differed, however, in being more precise in some goals and more generous in its funding. One section of Title V continued the requirement for single state agencies,[5] with a special division to direct maternal and child health and another division to direct crippled children's services. These divisions were usually placed in health departments. "Promoting the health of mothers and children" was understood to mean not only the supervision of maternity clinics and hospitals, but also the promotion of well-child conferences and the development of state capacity to monitor and promote maternal and child health.

Screening, as a federal policy goal, appeared in another section of Title V devoted to the care of crippled children. Its purpose was to enable each state to extend and improve

such state services for locating crippled children, and for providing medical, surgical, corrective, and other services and care, and facilities for diagnosis, hospitalization, and aftercare, for children who are crippled or who are suffering from conditions which lead to crippling. . . . (Section 511)

To locate such children, some sort of screening procedure was implied. Locating crippled children or children with conditions which might lead to crippling could have taken one of two forms: either a broadly conceived interpretation to set up state-wide screening procedures, or a more narrowly defined one to set up registries of crippled children. With the encouragement of the Children's Bureau, state officials chose the second form and created registries of crippled children. By 1945, the names of about 400,000 crippled children were reported to be on such registries.[6] However, the registries proved to be more activity reports on the Crippled Children's Program than reports on the health status of children, because they were not used for follow-up. Eventually, most states dropped the registries as being not very useful.

Thus, two types of screening developed from Title V: through MCH, the well-child conference; and through Crippled Children, registries of crippled children. Preventive care (primary prevention) was provided by the state and local maternal and child health services through supervision of maternity clinics, through nursing services for expectant mothers, through consultations with local health officials, and through the establishment of well-child conferences. Diagnosis and treatment were provided by the Crippled Children's Program, but only for those children with diseases covered by the program in that state. Services varied considerably from state to state. In the early days, they were mainly orthopedic, but later, diseases of the heart, cerebral palsy, cystic fibrosis, and others were added to the eligibility list. The Maternal and Child Health Program gave a small number of mothers and children medical and hospital care, but in the early years, the purpose was primarily to develop preventive services and to train personnel.[7]

The services provided under Title V increased in 1963 and again in 1965, when Congress authorized funds for projects for Maternity and Infant Care and for Children and Youth clinics. These programs sought to provide comprehensive care to children in targeted urban areas. For the first time a federal program brought together preventive and treatment services; but the mechanism, unlike that of the formula grants to state health departments mandated in 1935, was a system of projects in scattered sites across the United States. Each project was in itself intended to be comprehensive, but the program was not comprehensive for the United States as a whole.[8] The funding for Title V programs increased during these years. By 1970, the federal government was allocating $325 million for all Title V programs, both the state-wide formula grants and the projects (see table 1).

Thus, by the late 1960s there was a major functioning maternal and child health program, funded through grants to both state and health departments and localities, administered at the federal level first through the Children's Bureau and, after 1969, by the Public Health Service. These programs provided preventive and/or treatment services to about 7.5 percent of the country's children (see table 1).

States had wide latitude in the use of the formula grant MCH and CC funds. Later observers were to describe the system as an early form of revenue-sharing.[9] Nor was it clear that the matching funds each state was required to put up to receive federal funds represented new funds for child health. States often substituted federal funds for state funds, rather than use them as supplements.[10]

The Second Building Block: Medicaid (Title XIX)

Title XIX of the Social Security Act, or Medicaid as it became known, was not a program aimed specifically at children, but it rapidly became their largest public medical program after its establishment in 1966. By 1970, federal expenditures for children under Title XIX were $516 million compared to $223 million spent by the long-standing Title V programs. Medicaid served 9.4 percent of the child population in the United States (see table 1).

Unlike Title V, Medicaid grew out of the welfare system. It emerged as an afterthought in the passage of the Social Security Amendments of 1965, whose major contribution was the institution of a health insurance program for the elderly, Medicare.[11] The Medicaid program was intended to help public assistance recipients who were not covered by Medicare—that is, recipients of Aid to Families with Dependent Children (AFDC), Aid to the Blind (AB), and Aid to the Permanently and Totally Disabled (APTD). It would also supplement Medicare coverage for recipients of Old Age Assistance (OAA). The federal government would reimburse states through open-ended grants for some percentage (from 50 to 83 percent) of their actual expenditures. The exact federal match-

Table 1 Federal expenditures and services for children under twenty-one provided by Title V and Title XIX (Medicaid) of the Social Security Act (selected years)

	1940	1955	1970	1976
Federal Expenditures for Children under 21				
Title V	$8,058,000	$22,532,351	$223,504,648	$ 324,908,000[a]
Title XIX	—	—	$516,312,000	$1,457,625,000[b]
Number of Children Served				
Title V	1,698,529[c,d]	3,905,657[d]	6,074,675[e]	6,701,675[e]
Title XIX	—	—	7,614,000	11,053,000[f]
Percent of U.S. Population under 21 Served				
Title V	3.5	6.2	7.5	8.6
Title XIX	—	—	9.4	14.2

Sources:

Title V: Advisory Commission on Intergovernmental Operations, *Periodic Reassessment of Federal Grants-in-Aid to State and Local Governments* (Washington, D.C.: Government Printing Office, 1967) U.S., Department of the Treasury, *Annual Reports, Federal Aid to the States*, 1940, 1955, 1970. U.S., Department of Labor, *Services for Crippled Children Under the Social Security Act: Development of Program, 1936–39*, Children's Bureau Publication No. 258, 1941, table 12, p. 40; U.S., Department of Health, Education, and Welfare, *Maternal and Child Health Services in 1955*, Children's Bureau Statistical Series, no. 38, 1957, table B, p. 7; U.S., Department of Health, Education, and Welfare, *Maternal and Child Health Services of State and Local Health Departments, Fiscal Year 1970*, Maternal and Child Health Services (MCHS) Statistical Series No. 2, 1971, tables 7–9, 11; U.S., Department of Health, Education, and Welfare, *Maternal and Child Health Services of State and Local Health Department, Fiscal Years 1974, 1975, 1976*, MCHS Statistical Series no. 13, 1979, tables 7–10; U.S., Department of Health, Education, and Welfare, *Children Who Received Physician's Services Under the Crippled Children's Program, 1955*, MCHS Statistical Series, No. 3, 1955, table 1, and 1970, table 1. Unpublished data for 1976 (table 4) furnished by Edward Duffy, Bureau of Community Health Services, Department of Health, Education, and Welfare.

Title XIX: U.S., Department of Health, Education, and Welfare, *Number of Recipients and Amounts of Payments Under Medicaid, 1970*, NCSS, Report B–4 (1972), and unpublished data compiled for similar reports, 1976. U.S., Department of Health, Education, and Welfare, *Medicaid Management Reports, Annual Report, Fiscal Year 1976*, Medical Services Administration, table G.

Population: U.S., Department of Commerce, *Census of the Population*, 1940, 1970; U.S., Department of Commerce, *Statistical Abstract of the United States*, 1956, p. 32, 1977, p. 28.

[a] Represents funding levels, not expenditures.

[b] Estimated from total federal and state share.

[c] Data for 1940 were unavailable for crippled children, so 1939 figures were used to estimate the 1940 total.

[d] Maternal and child health services include infants and preschool children since the number of school children served was not reported.

[e] Special programs, immunizations, and dental treatment not included. Although all of these children were seen in Title V clinics, some of their services were financed by Title XIX. Therefore, these children appear in both Title V and XIX reports. There is no way of segregating these data.

[f] This number probably does not include the 1,743,396 children who received screening services during 1976. However, many of these children also received general Medicaid services as well. To add them would inflate the true number of children served.

ing percentages were calculated on the basis of a state's per capita income.[12]

As early as 1950, the federal government had reimbursed the states for a part of the medical expenses they chose to make on behalf of welfare clients. The states nonetheless were slow to participate in this program and expenditures for medical care rose only slowly.[13] It was not surprising therefore when, in 1965, the federal Commissioner of Welfare characterized medical services for AFDC children as "grossly inadequate."[14] The 1965 amendments were intended to increase both the quantity and quality of medical services available to welfare recipients.

Children were covered by Medicaid if their families qualified for AFDC by virtue of low income and the absence or unemployment of the father or if the children themselves were blind or disabled and thereby qualified for AB or APTD. The program also included a "medically needy" group of persons who did not receive cash payments because their family incomes were too high, but who were "categorically related" to the AFDC, AB, or APTD programs and whose medical expenses were high enough to require assistance. However, Senator Abraham Ribicoff of Connecticut thought this coverage was insufficient: "There are 5 million such children living in true poverty who cannot be aided under this bill because their father is living and is employed no matter how low his wages may be."[15] The Ribicoff amendment, which was accepted, allowed states at their option to be reimbursed by the federal government for medical assistance to all needy children under twenty-one. Need was defined according to income criteria only, and without regard to the children's categorical status.

All states choosing to participate in Medicaid were required to provide five basic services by 1967: in-patient hospital services, out-patient hospital services, laboratory services, skilled nursing home services for those over twenty-one, and physician services.[16] In addition, federal reimbursement was available to states choosing to provide a variety of optional services such as home health care, private duty nursing, clinic services, dental care, physical therapy, and prescribed drugs, dentures, and eyeglasses. Preventive care could also be paid for through Medicaid as part of the mandatory physician's services; however, data on preventive care visits was not routinely collected. One state welfare official, for example, said he had no information whatever on whether such services were actually provided.[17]

Eligibility

The Medicaid legislation as enacted established three categories of eligible children: those whose families received AFDC, AB, or APTD; the categorically related medically needy; and, by virtue of the Ribicoff amendment, children under twenty-one not in either of these two groups who were deprived of needed medical assistance because of low income. These three groups were known as the "categorically related," the "categorically related needy," and the "non-categorically related needy" respectively.[18]

Participating states were required to cover only the first category of children, those actually on welfare. However, those states electing to aid one or both of the other groups had to provide identical services to all eligible children. By 1971, all but two states had a Medicaid program. Twenty-five states offered medical assistance to the categorically related group in addition to recipients of AFDC, while only seventeen of the forty-eight participating states included the third category of financially eligible children under twenty-one.[19]

Income eligibility also varied widely among the states. In Oklahoma the maximum eligible income for a family of four was $2,448, while New York at its most generous provided medical assistance to comparable families earning $6,000.[20] Alarmed by rising costs, however, Congress included in the 1967 Social Security Amendments a provision limiting Medicaid reimbursement to payments for families with incomes no higher than 133⅓ percent of AFDC payment levels.[21] Thus, states like New York were forced to reduce their eligibility levels. Nevertheless, since AFDC grants varied from state to state, disparities in eligibility remained.[22]

As a result of these disparate eligibility requirements, the proportionate number of children receiving services also differed greatly among the states. In 1968, while New York aided 206 children per 1,000 inhabitants, South Carolina provided medical assistance to only 2 per 1,000.[23] By 1971, it was estimated that approximately ten million American children were eligible for Medicaid, seven million of whom were actually receiving services.[24] Had eligibility standards been applied uniformly throughout the United States at the level of the most generous states, and had financial rather than categorical need been the sole criterion, perhaps an additional ten to fifteen million children would have been eligible. Medicaid clearly had not brought all poor children into the "mainstream" of medical care.[25]

Financing and Services

Although the federal government bore part of Medicaid costs, the requirement of matching funds from the states constituted a disincentive to full participation. The richer, more populous states with the most extensive public health and welfare programs tended most fully to take advantage of the Medicaid program. In 1969, two states, New York and California, accounted for 45 percent of Medicaid expenditures.[26]

Despite this reluctance on the part of many states, Medicaid expenditures rose rapidly, from $2 billion in 1967 to $8.9 billion in 1973, and to $18 billion in 1978.[27] This increase reflected several factors: the number of states participating in Medicaid increased during this period from twenty-six to forty-nine; the cost of medical care, particularly of hospital care, rose sharply;[28] and the number of welfare recipients also increased.[29]

Medicaid quickly became the largest federal health program for children, both in expenditures and services; by 1970, it covered 9.4 percent of the nation's child population, while the Title V programs served only 7.5 percent. (See table 1 for a comparison of the Titles V and XIX programs.) Nevertheless, most Medicaid expenditures were on behalf of adults, who were the primary consumers of such expensive services as hospitalization and long-term convalescent care. More than 40 percent of Medicaid recipients were under twenty-one, but expenditures for children were only 15 percent of the program's budget in 1968 and 18 percent in 1971.[30]

Legacies of Titles V and XIX

By 1967, two major child health programs were functioning in the United States, both directed toward needy children. But whereas the Title V program attempted to be comprehensive, the Medicaid program was firmly tied to the means test. Title V addressed a health problem; Medicaid addressed a welfare problem.

The Title V program, particularly in its projects, provided preventive and treatment services to children. In other words, Title V attempted to serve comprehensively the children it reached, although it certainly reached only a small proportion of the poor children in the United States. Medicaid, on the other hand, was more comprehensive in its reach, at considerably greater cost, but less comprehensive in its services, with preventive care rarely being offered under the payment system.

A final major difference between the two programs lay in their administration. While Title V was directed in part to build and maintain state capacity to supervise maternal and child health care, Medicaid confined its efforts to paying providers for services rendered. The welfare departments or Title XIX agencies were merely pass-throughs and monitors for the appropriate disbursement of funds. They had no mandate to encourage utilization of services, and often discouraged it through red tape, low and delayed payments to providers, and slowness in ascertaining eligibility. While health departments had built some capacity to carry out maternal and child health planning, welfare departments learned to funnel funds to others, almost as fiscal agents.[31]

All the federal programs were to be directed toward children who lacked access to regular medical care. The Title V legislation of 1935 directed aid to areas suffering from "economic distress," or to rural areas where no care was available.[32] In 1943 Congress had at first rejected a request for funds for the Emergency Maternity and Infant Care (EMIC) Act because "there was no requirement of lack of financial ability as prerequisite to the benefits."[33] Only when Congress was reassured that the program was restricted to needy children by extending eligibility only to the four lowest pay grades in the armed services, did it appropriate the funds.

However, the Children's Bureau had been operating under a different philosophy. If it succeeded in avoiding a means test in the EMIC program, it was because it could reassure Congress that, at least, it would adhere to a restriction of eligibility by categories. As Sinai and Anderson point out: "The inclusion of a means test in the EMIC program would have meant a reversal of fundamental Bureau policy."[34] As early as 1926, one state official reported that their Bureau of Child Hygiene had been opening child health centers where children "of all classes" could be brought for free monthly examinations.[35] However, after World War II, the Children's Bureau philosophy of service to the whole community changed considerably. By the 1970s, means tests were being used in most states to assess eligibility for the Crippled Children's Program and in most aspects of the Maternal and Child Health Program as well. Nevertheless, the avoidance of a means test remained a part of federal administration philosophy in the Public Health Service. Even Maternity and Infant Care (MIC) and Children and Youth (C&Y) projects maintained they were willing to serve anyone who lived in the targeted community, but would set up a sliding fee schedule for those able to pay. Whether such a system actually avoids a means test is unclear, but its services were established and delivered before any means test was applied.

In contrast, Medicaid was tied directly to a means test as well as to categorical eligibility. One had to be found eligible before one could receive payment for medical services. These two contrasting traditions of Title V and Medicaid for providing child health services in the public sector were to influence the EPSDT legislation and provide considerable headaches in its implementation.

Beginnings of EPSDT [36]

By 1967, health services for needy children were being furnished by a number of different state and local agencies, in addition to the federal government. The various provider organizations—the American Academy of Pediatrics, committees of state medical societies, and the American Public Health Association—all tried to set standards for the care provided. No government program had yet attempted to provide preventive and treatment services in a comprehensive fashion. The time seemed ripe for a comprehensive plan for screening and treating children, most particularly those who did not receive care through the private sector.

Four major questions had to be resolved in the course of legislating, implementing, and administering such a program: (1) Which children were to be reached? (2) What quantity and quality of health services would be offered? (3) How much could/would be spent on the program? (4) Through what administering agency was the program to be implemented? The answer to the question of cost would, of course, affect decisions about the kind of care to be offered and the numbers of children to be reached. Because the planners of EPSDT did not address these issues systematically, the program was to create considerably more controversy during the years after it was signed into law than it did during its eight-month legislative gestation.

Federally sponsored periodic screening for low-income children was first mentioned in a 1966 Program Analysis prepared in the Office of the Secretary of HEW. These proposals were part of a series of systematic analyses developed to provide evaluation of ongoing programs and proposals for new programs for President Johnson's Great Society.[37] Three possible programs were suggested: a program serving an estimated one million newborns in health-depressed areas at a cost of approximately $30 million; another serving five million children living in health-depressed areas at birth and ages one, five, and nine at a cost of $150 million; and a third serving all the nation's 104,000 premature infants and costing a mere $5.3 million.[38] This was the only occasion where a federal document put a specific price tag on a specific nation-wide screening or preventive care program for specified child populations. It was suggested that the program "could be organized as an extension of the present Crippled Children's Program. Funds for such a program could come through the Title XIX 'Medicaid' program . . . ";[39] the document further proposed that Title XIX be amended to include diagnostic examinations. The seeds of administrative ambiguity were thus planted in this first report, perhaps because Title XIX was barely under way at the time the Program Analysis was written and its authors may have wanted to hedge their bets.[40] The document did not discuss in any detail the scope of services to be provided.

This study became the basis for President Johnson's child health initiatives. When he addressed Congress on 8 February 1967, he recommended that the existing appropriation for the care of needy children be doubled, for a total of $221 million, and that the number of needy children receiving care through the Crippled Children's Program be doubled to one million.[41] It was not clear, however, whether the increased funds and expanded services were intended for the same population.

Introduction of Legislation

Eight days later, Representative Wilbur Mills, following the president's lead, provided a small measure of clarification when he submitted legislation providing for a number of changes in the Social Security Act programs. The bill, known as H.R. 5710 or the Social Security Amendments of 1967, was described by the House Ways and Means Committee as including "revisions in the Old-Age, Survivors and Disability Insurance; provisions relating to health care for the aged and others (Title XVII and Title XIX); provisions relating to public assistance; tax provisions relating to senior citizens, etc."[42] Only those who already knew that nearly half the persons eligible for Title XIX were under twenty-one would have been alerted that a measure so described could affect children.

The EPSDT legislation within H.R. 5710 consisted of two amendments to Title XIX and one to Title V of the Social Security

Act. The major amendment to Title XIX, often referred to as the EPSDT amendment, was to provide

effective July 1, 1969, such early and periodic screening and diagnosis of individuals who are eligible under the plan and are under the age of 21—to ascertain their physical or mental defects, and such health care, treatment, and other measures to correct or ameliorate defects and chronic conditions discovered thereby, as may be provided in regulations of the Secretary. (Section 301(b)(1))

Only seven states specifically provided for such care in their state plans at the time the legislation was introduced;[43] its intent was to encourage the states to cover preventive services for children.

The other Title XIX amendment required that the state Title XIX agency enter into agreements with any agency receiving payment for part or all of its costs under Title V, use such an agency in furnishing care and services, and reimburse that agency for its services. The 1965 Medicaid legislation had similarly provided for the state Title XIX agencies to enter into agreements with the state agencies responsible for administering or supervising health services and vocational rehabilitation. EPSDT represented a departure from previous legislation in that the Title V agencies were specifically mentioned, the agreement was to include reimbursement, and the Secretary of HEW was to write regulations defining the scope of the relationship.[44]

The amendment to Title V provided that state health plans with regard to the Crippled Children's Program must

effective July 1, 1967, provide for early identification of children in need of health care and services, and for health care and treatment needed to correct or ameliorate defects or chronic conditions discovered thereby, through provision of such periodic screening and diagnostic services, and such treatment, care, and other measures to correct or ameliorate defects or chronic conditions as may be provided in regulations of the Secretary. (Section 301(a)(2))

This mandate to furnish preventive care replaced the weaker language of earlier provisions that required locating crippled children. The program's authorizations were to be increased from $55 to $65 million.[45] HEW's explanation of the act's provisions stated that the amendment to Title XIX plus the "proposed increase of $15 million [sic] in the authorization for 'Crippled Children's Services' and the requirement . . . that such services include periodic screening and diagnosis would greatly strengthen the nation's programs for children."[46] This document did not, however, indicate how the program was to be administered nor how many children were to be served.

Hearings on H.R. 5710 were held before the House Ways and Means Committee in March and April 1967. The revised bill, known as H.R. 12080 when it emerged from the Ways and Means Committee in August 1967, was discussed in Senate Finance Committee hearings during August and September of the same year. During each of these three stages of the EPSDT program's early legislative history, the issues of cost and administration were taken up, while scope of services and eligible population were more frequently ignored.

First Public Discussion: H.R. 5710 Hearings

Comment on the child health amendments constituted only a small part of the nearly three thousand pages of testimony on H R 5710, and most of that concerned costs rather than any of the other three issues that would determine the shape of the future program. The witnesses, however, seemed confused as to whether Title V or Title XIX was to foot the bill. HEW had suggested that an additional $100 million, earmarked for children, be authorized for Title XIX and an extra $15 million for Crippled Children be added to the Title V appropriation; some part of the Title XIX money was intended for expansion of all the states' services to children, not only preventive care.[47] George Meany welcomed the President's proposals for "an increase of $100 million in federal financial participation for needy children," but added the amounts authorized for child health were the "absolute minimum required."[48] The American Parents' Committee[49] and the American Academy of Orthopedic Surgeons,[50] presumably referring to the Crippled Children authorization, supported the $10 million increase to cover additional case finding and increased medical costs. Other organizations, however, were less sure that the amounts requested were sufficient to meet the increased costs anticipated; the American Cerebral Palsy Association stated that an extra $18 million was needed.[51] The Foundation for the Blind[52] and the State of Illinois Commission on Children[53] both objected that the CC program's closed-ended funding would limit the kinds of services that could be provided; Title XIX funding, by contrast, is open-ended. The strongest request for additional support for the CC program came from the organization of those who administered it, the Association of State and Territorial Health Officers.

Their testimony stated that, due to a 1965 law requiring the CC program to pay "reasonable cost" for hospital services, the "greatly increased cost is working a tremendous hardship in these programs . . . "; without the provision of additional federal funds "there is every possibility that [these increased costs] will result in a reduced amount of care given.[54]

This uncertainty about the funding of the new program reflected an underlying confusion about whether the program was Title V or Title XIX, health or welfare, and which of the two preceding traditions was to prevail. HEW Secretary Gardner called for agreements between the Title XIX and Title V (Crippled Children) agencies,[55] while Martha M. Eliot, former head of the Children's Bureau, "heartily" approved of this relation.[56] The American Nursing Association stated that the purpose of the legislation was to broaden the base of the Children's Bureau Title V programs, and ignored the role of the Title XIX agency.[57] Congressman James A. Burke of Massachusetts made the only comment on the ambiguity, saying: "It is a program that should be administered by the Department of Public Health. . . . It is not a welfare program. It is a health program."[58] The fundamental issue of whether health or welfare departments should pay for and implement a health program for welfare children was not resolved during these or subsequent hearings, and continued to plague all those charged with implementing the program.

Questions of eligibility for and scope of the proposed program likewise received scant attention, and produced conflicting points of view. In accord with the president's suggestion, Secretary Gardner proposed that 500,000 additional children be screened during the first year of operation, and that within three to five years the program be extended to five million children; he did not specify whether these children were to be served through Crippled Children or the Title XIX program.[59] The American Parents' Committee also endorsed this 500,000 figure, assuming that case finding would take place within the context of the CC program, although the target population was low-income or medically indigent children.[60]

Eligibility for the new program was also a matter of some uncertainty. Some witnesses felt that state CC services ought to expand to include children with vision or hearing problems. Others voiced concern that some specialized services of the CC program might no longer be available to the working poor if the Medicaid eligibility criteria became the sole criterion for receiving services. These ambiguities also were not resolved prior to the law's enactment.

The hearings produced virtually no discussion of the scope and extent of screening and preventive and follow-up care to be carried out; these details were to be prescribed by the Secretary of HEW.

Phase 2—H.R. 12080

The three EPSDT amendments remained essentially unchanged when the 1967 Social Security amendments were reported out of the Ways and Means Committee as H.R. 12080. The program was, however, indirectly affected by the many major changes in the Social Security Act.[61] For example, the committee's bill consolidated all Title V funding into one authorization of $250 million, of which the MCH services and CC services were to receive a total of $125 million; if this sum were divided equally between the two programs, CC would receive an authorization of $62.5 million, a few million dollars less than had been proposed in H.R. 5710.[62]

The proposed effective date of the Title V amendment, 1 July 1967, had already passed and was therefore deleted; 1 July 1969 remained as the effective date of the Title XIX amendment. The EPSDT amendment to Title V had been written into a new consolidated Title V, and the two Title XIX amendments labeled "conforming amendments."[63]

The Ways and Means Committee's report appeared to meet the question of administrative authority for the program, emphasizing that the EPSDT provisions were to result in more aggressive casefinding by the CC program. The committee then obscured its intent, however, by suggesting that other programs would also find cases:

Organized and intensified case-finding procedures will be carried out in well baby clinics, day care centers, nursery schools, Headstart centers in cooperation with the Office of Economic Opportunity, by periodic screening of children in schools, through follow-up visits by nurses to the homes of newborn infants, by checking birth certificates for the reporting of congenital malformation and by related activities. Title XIX (Medical Assistance) would be modified to conform to this requirement under the formula grant program.[64]

Although the legislation affected only the CC and Title XIX programs, the committee was suggesting that all other federal, state, and local programs be asked to cooperate as well, despite the absence of either funding or an administrative framework for such an endeavor. The report did not mention that much of the screening ongoing at that time was in fact supported by the MCH program.

The committee report proposed that EPSDT be administered through the CC program, although case finding would also be carried out under the Title XIX program; the Title XIX agency was expected to provide reimbursement to the Title V agency.[65] CC's authorization was increased by only $7.5 million to fund this massively expanded program, an amount that by itself was unlikely to bring about increased services by the states' MCH and CC agencies. The amount of Title XIX money to be available for EPSDT was not specified, but the federal open-ended funding of Title XIX gave that program greater flexibility.

Finally, the committee mentioned neither the number of children to be reached by this expanded program nor the extent of services to be provided. The House passed H.R. 12080 in August and sent it to the Senate with the fundamental issues concerning EPSDT—cost, eligible population, extent of care, and method of administration—still not clarified. The latter two questions were explicitly delegated to the Secretary of HEW to determine by regulation. The Senate's hearings cast no greater light on what Congress intended the legislation to do.

Phase 3—Senate Hearings and Passage
The Senate Finance Committee held hearings on H.R. 12080 during August and September 1967. Since the EPSDT provisions had been left unchanged by the House Ways and Means Committee, the program received little attention. Only one witness, Dr. Donald C. Smith of the American Academy of Pediatrics, stressed the need for preventive health measures in childhood and asked that the high quality of the CC program be maintained. He recommended an amendment that would require cooperation between state agencies administering their CC programs and those administering Title XIX programs.[66] Congress, however, retained the more ambiguous existing wording that directed state Title XIX agencies to provide for "entering into agreements" with Title V and other agencies.

The lack of concern about EPSDT seems odd in that these hearings dealt extensively with restricting the costs of Medicaid, which this new program would greatly increase. Perhaps EPSDT's proponents, aware of its high potential cost and also of the jurisdictional dispute it could provoke between health and welfare agencies, deliberately underplayed these problem areas. The three amendments constituting the EPSDT program were passed by the Senate without change, and as part of PL 90–248 were signed into law by President Johnson on 2 January 1968.

EPSDT was the first federal policy mandating preventive health services for needy children—a kind of health insurance for the poor. It required states with Title XIX programs [67] to provide such services for all eligible children. In addition, the CC program would also have to include early periodic screening for its eligible population. The breadth of this legislative mandate was clear; the program's specifics remained obscure. The Office of the Secretary of HEW would find little guidance for writing regulations which could translate legislative intent into a viable program.

Regulations and Guidelines

The EPSDT legislation stipulated that it be implemented by 1 July 1969; however, final regulations and guidelines did not appear for four and one-half years after the bill became law. Proposed regulations were issued in December 1970, final regulations appeared in November 1971, and final guidelines in June 1972; final implementation for all age groups was deferred until 1 July 1973. Throughout this four and one-half year period HEW held extensive discussions as to the direction rule-making should take. The participants were numerous—administrators and planners for the Title V and Title XIX programs in Washington, individual congressmen and senators and Congress as a whole, the state Title XIX and Title V agencies (generally the welfare and health departments), the HEW regional offices, the National Welfare Rights Organization (NWRO), the Medical Assistance Advisory Council (MAAC), and professional groups such as the American Optometric Association. HEW became the battleground for issues which had not been resolved during the program's legislative history, but which had to be clarified before regulations and guidelines could be published and the program implemented.

Administering Agency

The legislation never clarified whether EPSDT was to be administered through Title XIX or by the Title V (Crippled Children's) program. During the summer of 1968, HEW Secretary Wilbur Cohen delegated the job of developing regulations, not to the Maternal and Child Health Services (MCHS) which administered CC, but rather to the Medical Services Administration (MSA). Writing regulations was a new procedure for MSA. Prior to 1968, Title XIX programs had provided all guiding material to the states through its *Handbook of Medical Assistance—Supplement D*. Since these guidelines gave no way for the public or interested parties to be heard, and since several different agencies had been placed together during the 1968 reorganization of HEW, their policies had to be standarized and regulations had to be written. H.R. 12080 required that regulations be written for use of skilled nursing homes as well as for EPSDT, and both these regulations were several years aborning. In consultation with Dr. Arthur Lesser, the MCHS director, MSA developed an administrative strategy for the program whereby the state Title XIX and Title V agencies would make firm agreements with one another. Using MCHS personnel as consultants, MSA proceeded to draft regulations and take on the role of administrator for the EPSDT program.

After proposed EPSDT regulations were published in December 1970, states began to question whether the Title V or XIX agencies could cooperate and how they could avoid duplicating one another's efforts.[68] The Medicaid program was to provide for "identification of those eligible individuals who are in need of medical or remedial care and services furnished through Title V grantees, and for assuring that such individuals are informed of such services and are referred to Title V grantees for proper care and services, as appropriate."[69] Neither Congress nor HEW had considered that these health and welfare agencies might not work well together on the state level. MCHS wanted the guidelines to spell out the relationship in greater detail, while state and regional officials questioned why other relevant organizations, such as home health agencies, had not been mentioned.

The major source of conflict and confusion in this interagency relationship proved to be the question of reimbursement. Early in 1970, MSA had requested a legal opinion on what the regulations required. The ruling stated that the Title V agency was entitled to total reimbursement for all services furnished; further, the Title XIX agency was not entitled to control over the number of children screened nor to the amounts reimbursed except as provided in the written agreements, and reimbursement could not be limited to children referred by the Title XIX agency. But the state Title XIX agencies were reluctant to abide by this ruling, perhaps because it required payment for services which had hitherto been furnished by the Title V agencies at no charge to the recipients. The following year MSA slightly weakened its stand, ruling that payment by the Title XIX agencies could include both diagnostic and treatment services "as appropriate," and noting that allocating responsibility for payment was a matter of program policy rather than a legal question. The reimbursement issue was particularly difficult to resolve because in many states the Title V programs were the major providers of public screening, diagnostic, and treatment services through the CC program. Because their funding had not been increased they were having considerable trouble maintaining their programs, and consequently pursued vigorously the possibility of reimbursement through EPSDT. The Title XIX agencies, on the other hand, were under considerable pressure from state governments hard hit by inflation to cut expenditures, and therefore resisted these demands for payment for Title V services. Despite MSA's efforts to force the state agencies to work out their own relationships, they continued to appeal to their respective HEW agencies for support, requiring MSA to reiterate its position on reimbursement in a memorandum issued the following year.

Between 1968 and 1972, MSA emerged as the primary administrator of the EPSDT program, while MCHS acted mainly as a consultant; by 1973, MSA was awarding contracts for EPSDT program evaluations and development of screening standards. MCHS, however, was not entirely pleased with MSA's move into the field of health services, and this tension at the federal level was reflected within the state agencies. It is not clear whether the lack of harmony at the state level was encouraged by the MSA-MCHS rivalry, or whether the state agencies were simply not amenable to control from above; one MSA administrator was unsure whether MSA at this time had a policy of encouraging inter-agency relations, since the guidelines did not reflect any. The ever-present question of reimbursement between the two agencies constantly brought these tensions to the surface, with the state agencies attempting to involve their federal counterparts in the dispute. The fundamental ambiguity of the program's administrative structure thus was painfully apparent to all those charged with its implementation.

Costs and Funding

Making EPSDT a Title XIX program determined its financing. Since Medicaid's funding is open-ended, with the federal government reimbursing the states for 50 to 83 percent of their expenditures, theoretically there were no limits on the development of EPSDT programs; however, prosperous states like California and New York had taken advantage of the Title XIX program, while the smaller, poorer states had not. Further, when states had spent a great deal of money, as had New York and California at the inception of Medicaid, Congress objected that costs were too high.[70]

According to MSA and state officials, the data available on the projected cost of EPSDT were so poor that estimates were not made for the first two years after the program's enactment. By August 1970, however, it had been suggested that operation for the first year would cost $45 million, a sum so alarming that HEW delayed issuing regulations because of EPSDT's "great cost" to both federal and state governments. The agency requested that the program be phased in gradually,[71] but Congress refused. Meanwhile, Senator Abraham Ribicoff and the MAAC continued to press for regulations.

When proposed regulations were published, eighteen out of the twenty-two states submitting comments stated that the program would impose a financial burden beyond the states' capacity; one southern state had its entire congressional delegation send letters voicing alarm. The federal guidelines were still not available, however, so that the states could not estimate costs with any accuracy.[72]

During the spring of 1971, the Nixon Administration committed itself to reducing federal Medicaid costs for fiscal 1972. The administration was at the time proposing the ill-fated Family Health Insurance Plan (FHIP) and EPSDT was held up while HEW studied how they fit together. Officials in the Secretary's office even considered getting legislation to eliminate EPSDT altogether. HEW followed this lead by announcing that the states would be permitted to implement EPSDT in phases, beginning with children under six, in order to soften the impact on state budgets, which would of course lessen the federal government's costs as well. HEW officials were still worried, however, that EPSDT's costs would be excessive, with one estimate of $400 million by 1973. As a result, HEW decided to narrow the scope of services, and slowly to phase in successive age groups. In September 1971, the agency submitted a first-year cost of only $25 million; approval of this sum by the Office of Management and Budget permitted final regulations to be published.

Thus, the states had delayed for nearly three years implementation of a duly enacted statute.[73] Because their commitment to the federal policy was insufficient, and/or because their financial situation was sufficiently pressing, the states did their utmost to hinder implementation. HEW, caught between the congressional proponents of EPSDT and the state welfare agencies who were its clients, temporized by permitting the states to phase in the program gradually.

Eligibility

The eligibility issue was resolved when EPSDT became a Title XIX program, since any child who was eligible under the state Medicaid plan became eligible for EPSDT. However, as noted earlier, state plans varied considerably in their eligibility requirements, resulting in tremendous national disparities. In all, an estimated ten million children, or 12 percent of the child population, were eligible for EPSDT in 1968. The states were permitted initially to restrict eligibility for the program to children under six, with older children to be served by 1973; despite the explicitly temporary nature of this limitation, however, some states in fact were very slow to phase in the over-six population.

Scope of Services

From the outset, it was assumed that the services offered by the EPSDT program were to be comprehensive in all respects, and this thinking was reflected in the proposed regulations published in 1970:

Effective January 1, 1971 (or earlier at the option of the State), that early and periodic screening and diagnosis to ascertain physical and mental defects, and treatment of conditions discovered *regardless of the limits otherwise imposed under the State plan* on the type and amount of such care and services . . . will be available to all eligible individuals under 21 years of age.[74]

The forty-eight states operating Medicaid programs at the time varied widely in the scope of services offered. Only Minnesota provided the full range of services for which federal reimbursement was available, while others offered only a few in addition to the five mandatory services. Dental care and eyeglasses were excluded in eighteen states, and prescription drugs in eight.[75] To assure comprehensive care, the federal regulations would necessarily have to disregard the limits of state plans.

Not surprisingly, the states objected vigorously, claiming that the regulations contravened the intent of Title XIX and federal-state grant programs in general because they deprived the states of control over the scope of their programs. Some state officials also argued that existing medical manpower was not sufficient to carry out such a comprehensive program. They also suggested that periodic screening was an outmoded concept largely abandoned by public health and medical personnel.

Strong support for the regulations came from the director of the National Legal Program on Health Problems of the Poor, who also effectively lobbied other groups, particularly welfare rights groups, to enlist their support for EPSDT. He asked that the regulations specify the particular services covered, such as eyeglasses, hearing aids, and dental fillings.

The mounting concern about EPSDT's cost at both the state and federal levels resulted in a retreat from MSA's original position on the scope of services under EPSDT; the final regulations required the states to provide care "within the limits of the state plan on the amount, duration and scope of care and services."[76] Although this represented a severe cutback of the treatment offered under EPSDT, the welfare rights lobby had at least succeeded in including in the regulations the requirement that regardless of its plan a state had to provide "eyeglasses, hearing aids, and other kinds of treatment for visual and hearing defects, and at least such dental care as is necessary for relief of pain and infection and for restoration of teeth and maintenance of dental health. . . ." These three treatment services, together with early and periodic screening, thus constituted the EPSDT program as embodied in the final regulations.

Through its guidelines MSA tried to encourage the states to develop the most comprehensive programs possible. MCHS made available the expertise that agency had developed on child health services. In addition, groups such as the American Optometric Association voiced the interests of their own professions, asking that specific care such as visual screening and restorative services be included. The final guidelines reflecting these influences described case-finding procedures, screening tests to be performed, and diagnosis, treatment, and therapeutic services to be made available to eligible children.[77] It should be stressed, however, that the guidelines were advisory and that the services to be carried out in any particular state depended on the provisions of its Medicaid plan.

Those who had viewed EPSDT as a major innovative comprehensive health program for needy children found the regulations a disappointment. Those with a "toe-in-the-door" philosophy of federal policy-making, however, found it an encouraging first step. EPSDT unquestionably expanded the scope of services available to poor children; in fact, one state official commented that the same services were not always available to middle-income children.

2 *Implementation*

Congressional Neglect

As the preceding legislative and regulatory history indicates, Congress had paid very little attention to the law it had just passed. True, it had established for the first time a program to provide preventive care and follow-up treatment for poor children eligible for Medicaid. However, it had not laid out much rationale for this program and the principle of comprehensive health care for poor children was not discussed in its debates. More important, the issues of cost, scope of services, and administering agency were left sufficiently vague that implementation of such a massive principle was clearly not what Congress had in mind. The statement of principle was made almost invisible by the absence of supporting documentation and allocations.

Once having enacted the law, Congress then showed downright neglect. The law had never been the project of any one congressman and thus no one chose to oversee it. When HEW failed to issue regulations, only Representative William F. Ryan and Senator Ribicoff applied any pressure at all, and the latter did not press very hard.[78] At one point in 1972, when the law was already to have taken effect, the Senate Finance Committee voted to postpone for two years the requirement that states provide screening services for children over six and to remove the burden of the regulations already published which required them to provide visual, hearing, and dental treatment for defects discovered.[79] However, by the time the committee had issued its report, it had taken a 180 degree turn and not only reiterated its original stand of requiring implementation, but also required that a 1 percent penalty be applied to the AFDC funds of any state which failed to seek out and inform potential recipients of the availability of the program. The change had occurred with as little explanation and as much of a political compromise as the original legislation. The only explanation was in a brief paragraph.[80] In fact, until the moment that the amendment was passed, most congressmen assumed that EPSDT was to be scrapped. Instead, it survived with more obligations.

For the next five years, congressional involvement with the ambiguous law it had created took the form of pot shots at HEW for failure to codify and implement what it itself had been unable to clarify. Committee hearings, General Accounting Office reports, and the *Congressional Record* served as the forums for these outbursts.[81] At one point, a congressional committee accused HEW of "maladministration" leading to "crippling, retardation, and even death of hundreds of thousands of children."[82] Congress seemed unable to understand that the reasons for these alleged failures lay as much in the structure of the law as in bureaucratic obstinacy.

HEW's Neglect

Congressional attacks upon HEW and the bureaucracy were not entirely unjustified. HEW proved no better than Congress at making its policy clear. Since EPSDT was and is a federal-state program, and since the screening requirement was something new for the states, successful implementation required strong guidance from Washington. Unfortunately, this never materialized. The history of EPSDT in HEW was characterized by a vacillating policy reflected by uncertain goals, the low allocation of resources for program administration, and decentralization.

HEW suffered severe internal problems in setting its priorities during this period. The EPSDT program had been sponsored and passed by a Democratic president. However, his Secretary of HEW had not published regulations during the following year. When a Republican, President Nixon, took office in 1969, the regulations were delayed for another three years.

Vacillating policy was most reflected in the history of HEW's lack of enforcement of the 1972 penalty regulations, which will be discussed more fully in part II. It suffices to say here that regulations for this amendment were not published until 1974, one month after they were to have taken effect. The first states were cited for penalties a year later, but by the end of 1980, no penalties had actually been applied. Meanwhile, the regulations had been changed and several attempts had been made by administrations to change the legislation and have the penalties eliminated. The result was a continuing policy of vacillation with states able to resist successfully federal demands for program compliance. The one enforcing tool which Congress had made available to HEW was not used effectively by that agency because of its own uncertain goals.

Meanwhile, because of external pressure, HEW had been obliged to upgrade EPSDT as a major concern and high priority. The outside pressures came from advocacy groups that had filed suits against the welfare departments for failure to carry out the program. Between 1972 and 1976, such suits were filed in fifteen states, and the decisions, when handed down, tended to favor the plaintiffs.[83] For the states to accede to court demands, they needed help from HEW. Other pressures were applied directly to HEW. These included in 1974 an article in the *National Journal* and a TV program condemning HEW. HEW reacted by having senior officials claim that EPSDT was a high priority,[84] and by listing EPSDT as the first of a list of priorities in an HEW report entitled *Understanding Medicaid*.[85] In a reply to a critical report of the House Oversight and Investigations Subcommittee, the administrator of the Social and Rehabilitation Services, under whose aegis Medicaid functioned, defended the program by acknowledging that "the Department and the States were not initially responsive to the opportunities and responsibilities of the EPSDT program. . . . It is also true, however, that the program has been a major HEW priority since 1974."[86]

If, as those at HEW's highest level claimed, EPSDT was a high priority, this was not always visible from the way it allocated its resources. HEW had often been unwilling to budget sufficient funds to implement its Medicaid programs. Staffing was a particular problem. By 1972, Medicaid, which paid out a total of $6.7 billion in federal and state funds, had, in Washington, an authorized staff of only two hundred persons.[87] Four years later the outlay of funds had more than doubled to $14.7 billion, but the number of staff in Washington was still about two hundred.[88]

As a subdivision of the Medicaid program, EPSDT depended on this same system. However, the EPSDT program required administrative tasks which were far beyond Medicaid's scope. Under EPSDT, HEW had to see that states could identify eligible children, and that they sought out and informed parents of the program. They had to make sure that states followed up children who needed additional care. They had to assure that standards for care were set and that they were appropriate. They had to monitor that the amount of care rendered to the population was appropriate. Such reporting was not necessary under Medicaid as a whole, which functioned basically to pay bills, not to assure that people received needed care. Moreover, the EPSDT program had to maintain liaison with other HEW bureaus or other federal agencies which also provided child health care.

Despite EPSDT's greater administrative complexity and despite statements that EPSDT was a priority for HEW, staffing was low and erratic. Between 1972 and 1974 a small staff devoted to EPSDT monitoring was built up, but by early summer 1974, under HEW Secretary Caspar Weinberger's "cost-saving" and efficiency restrictions, Medicaid and EPSDT administrative morale had declined; monitoring staff had been cut back to the point that only two persons familiar with the EPSDT program remained. Then, external pressure in 1974 caused a dedicated administrative staff to be gradually built up again under the supervision of a socially concerned director, Beatrice Moore. The program was first a subdivision within the monitoring unit of the Medical Services Administration (MSA); later, in the spring of 1975, it became one of the eight divisions of MSA. However, it never achieved a professional staff of more than about twenty persons despite the many tasks which were assigned to it, and even as late as 1977 the Medicaid director was wondering whether he had made the right decision in setting up a separate division.[89] When HEW was reorganized in 1978, the EPSDT unit was moved out from under Medicaid and given separate status as the Office of Child Health in the Health Care Financing Administration (HCFA). However, the staff did not increase and there was therefore some question whether the staff, despite its dedication to the program, could handle increased assignments.[90]

Administrative changes in higher levels of HEW, a planned move from Washington to Baltimore, a scarcity of staff, and, finally, the charge by HEW Secretary Joseph Califano that the leadership failure lay within the Office of Child Health, caused morale within the unit to plummet again. As one devoted program administrator commented: "With the landscape heaving the way it is, it's hard not to feel a little nauseous." As a result, by early 1979 that office retained only one senior person who had worked on the program for more than a few months. Without an institutional memory, policy continued to vacillate. HEW could neither set a good example for its programs, nor guide state policy. As an earlier HEW report had noted, "At worst, screening services can become another fragmented health service. While this is not the intent of EPSDT, lack of guidance by the federal government to the program in early years has exacerbated the situation."[91]

In September 1977, Congress had held hearings on improvements for the EPSDT program. At that time Representative Paul Rogers, Chairman of the House Subcommittee on Health and the Environment, requested Secretary Califano to produce within thirty days information for Congress on the administration of EPSDT and its potential successor, the Child Health Assessment Program (CHAP).[92]

Work had begun on two such reports and proceeded slowly. One report focused on the administration of EPSDT itself and its potential successor, CHAP; the other report examined the relations of the EPSDT/CHAP office with other HEW offices.[93] Both emphasized the special position and administrative needs of the EPSDT program within HEW and within the Medicaid program.

Although both reports circulated within HEW for some time, and although some of their recommendations became the basis for administrative changes, neither was ever officially accepted by Secretary Califano, nor sent to Congress. This constituted another in the long series of instances of congressional neglect and HEW inconstancy.

A third area of problems for the HEW bureaucracy in enforcing its policy resulted from an extra bureaucratic layer between HEW in Washington and the states. Under the Nixon Administration, the ten HEW regional offices had been given greater autonomy with respect to Washington. This decentralization scheme had left central Medicaid offices without line authority over regional office staff and resulted in the regional offices occasionally seeming to be spokesmen more for the states than for the federal government. These attitudes showed up in the penalty reviews undertaken by the regional offices. In some regions, strict criteria were followed. In other regions, the criteria were less stringent so that states with similar implementation problems in one region would be assessed for the penalty and in another would not, depending upon the criteria of the regional office.[94]

Thus, the layering of bureaucracy gave an additional element of uncertainty to the federal policy. HEW's vacillating policy toward EPSDT was evident from the law's enactment, right on through the 1970s. That this was a period which saw four presidential administrations only illustrates more clearly that the vacillation was intrinsic to HEW, not necessarily to the presidents who came and went. It may also illustrate an important lesson about the persistence of executive non-policy despite changes in administrations.

If an executive agency is determined not to follow a policy, it can do so through Democratic and Republican administrations, and through changes of Congress. Persistence of policy, often described as a problem in governmental relations, seems to have been characteristic of EPSDT policy; that is, persistence of inconstancy was part of the governmental ethos.

Resolving Ambiguities: The States Have a Try

With congressional neglect and HEW uncertainty, it was not surprising that the states moved slowly to carry out the federal mandate. They had been among the first to notice EPSDT's potential costs, and were having enough trouble dealing with Medicaid as a whole.[95] To carry out EPSDT the states would have to resolve the major issues left ambiguous in the legislation and the regulations: administering agency, eligibility, services to be delivered. and costs.

To discuss EPSDT as a national program is difficult because the assessment of each state's performance has to take into account the rules by which each state was operating. To administer and monitor EPSDT were equally difficult because of the multiplicity of standards and criteria. For all these differences, there are several common and recurrent patterns in the states' responses to the program.

Eligibility

The 1971 regulations set eligibility qualifications: EPSDT would cover any child eligible under the state's Medicaid program. However, this represented a patchwork of eligibility determinations which varied from state to state. The states had first to estimate how many of its children were eligible. Those states which covered only those children on welfare (AFDC) could do this with relative ease, since they kept case files on each family and rechecked eligibility frequently. However, states which included the medically needy and the financially eligible found it harder to make estimates, since the children came to the attention of Medicaid agencies only when they or their families had some pressing medical need.[96] Usually Medicaid agencies were alerted by hospitals waiting to be paid for a service for which the child had no coverage. In 1973, when states were first required to report, 9.7 million children were estimated to be eligible for screening, diagnosis, and treatment under EPSDT.[97] Thus, at the minimum, 12 percent of the child population of the United States became potentially eligible for preventive care. However, the true number of children eligible remained throughout the program a mysterious floating estimate. State officials were also not above deflating the estimates when it became clear that their performance in getting children screened was going to be measured against the total number of children eligible.[98] Nor was it sufficient for states to estimate the number eligible at any one time; they also had to take into account the number who became eligible at any time during the year. Since children (and their parents) went on and off AFDC and other eligibility rolls during the year, a formula was worked out in the early days whereby the number of children during the year was calculated as being 1.3 times the number eligible at one time. After 1976, when HEW officials concluded that the turnover in the AFDC rolls was not as great as originally expected, they deflated the figure to 1.2.

Administration

The states administered Medicaid variously by the welfare or social service agency, the health department, an umbrella agency which included both health and welfare, or in one state, Mississippi, by an independent commission. In twenty-seven states, the welfare agency was the legally designated Medicaid agency; in fifteen states and in Washington, D.C., this task was undertaken by an umbrella agency. In some states this umbrella agency represented an integration of health and welfare departments; in others it was a true umbrella agency, in which the health and welfare departments remained functionally separate with Medicaid assigned to the welfare section. Only six states assigned Medicaid to the health department.[99]

The significance of this distribution of administrative responsibilities in the states lay in the fact that EPSDT required a combination of provider enrollment, bill payment, outreach, follow-up, and standard-setting for health care. Welfare agencies had not needed these skills for administering Medicaid; health agencies were more likely to have developed them. To overcome their insufficiency, some state welfare departments contracted with health departments to have them either carry out the screening, do the outreach, or both. States such as Michigan and Texas contracted with the health departments to carry out all screening services under the program. Other states, such as Vermont, contracted with the health department to contact and inform children of the availability of screening services, while reimbursing a variety of providers for screening services. Health and welfare departments often had trouble working together. The relationship between health and welfare agencies seemed to work best and produce the highest rates of service in states where there was a history of cooperative relationships between the two departments and where each department was well staffed and well organized.[100]

Aside from the skills needed to manage a health program, general administrative skills were required to oversee the information systems to run a program that included varying eligibility criteria and the responsibility to seek out and inform people that services were available.

Not only did state governments lack skills, they lacked as well interest in undertaking the new program. This was reflected in the staffing patterns. If HEW had trouble staffing Medicaid, the same could be said for the states. Administrative costs were kept low: in the various states only an average of 4 percent of total federal and state Medicaid funds were expended for administration.[101] Each state designated an EPSDT coordinator, who was duly listed in HEW publications. In some states this person might spend all his time on EPSDT; in other states he might spend as little as 10 percent of his time on the program. States had frequent hiring freezes, which would limit the staff that could be specifically added for a new program such as EPSDT.[102]

The administrative problems experienced by the states mirrored those of the federal government: limited staff and limited skills. But the states had the more difficult tasks to perform. While the federal agency only had to oversee the states' performance, the states had to deliver the services. States had to identify children in need, arrange for providers of services, reach the children, assure follow-up, and maintain records. This last requirement was most difficult of all for many states. Although, during this period, 90 percent federal matching grants encouraged states to install computerized systems which would allow them to monitor more closely the flow of funds, and search out fraud and abuse under Medicaid, the states were very slow to install such systems. By 1977, only twelve states had certified operating Medicaid Management Information Systems. Two years later, the number had risen to only twenty-five states.[103] Moreover, since the planning for these systems had begun before EPSDT was implemented, they usually lacked the appropriate software for assessing EPSDT performance.

It proved difficult, as well, to mobilize administrative resources for a program which state legislatures did not ardently desire. After all, it was a federal mandate, not a state one. Moreover, unlike a number of other Medicaid programs which had been introduced, EPSDT could not result in the states simply being able to collect federal matching funds for services they had already been providing through their own funds. EPSDT required new services for children who had not previously been reached. In no way would it be cheap. Any attempt to extend staff and carry out a search for the eligible children would simply generate a demand for services which many states were not willing to undertake.

Services

Despite the federal requirement that states begin the EPSDT program by 7 February 1972, and implement it state-wide by 1 July 1973, only twenty-eight states had begun implementation by the first date, and by the second date only thirty-two states had a state-wide program.[104] Ohio, for example, did not even begin a pilot program until September 1973 and was not carrying out the program throughout the state until 1974, well after the required starting dates.[105] States had three problems in providing services: they had to determine what screening services they would pay for; they had to find providers of those services; and they had to identify and inform children (or their parents) that they were eligible for these services

Few, if any, states had paid for screening or preventive services under Medicaid. Some states, such as Connecticut, claimed they did, but this proved impossible to document. Fortunately, HEW had carefully defined what screening meant in guidelines published in June 1972.[106] These guidelines defined screening as

the use of quick simple procedures carried out among large groups of people to sort out apparently well persons from those who have a disease or abnormality and to identify those in need of more definitive study of their physical or mental problems.[107]

They suggested nineteen screening procedures, including the taking of a health history; an unclothed physical assessment including physical growth; assessment of nutritional and immunization status; developmental assessment; ear, nose, mouth, and throat inspection; testing of vision, hearing, and urine; and tests for anemia, sickle cell, tuberculosis, and lead poisoning. Most states adopted most of these recommendations for their own programs.[108] Several states with very small black populations omitted sickle cell testing. This decision made a certain amount of sense, but why other states omitted certain procedures such as lead poisoning screening or assessment of nutritional status was not always clear. Little information is available on how the states determined what would be in the screening package. It is evident that most states relied on the federal guidelines, but except for those states in which health departments became actively involved in the screening or advising, state welfare departments for the most part determined the acceptable tests and based them on the federal recommendations.

Two problems arose. First, many states felt that where private physicians did the screening they should not be required to carry out all the same procedures as health department screening clinics. However, HEW made it clear that private physicians had to provide equivalent services.[109] Second, states disagreed over how often a child should be seen between birth and the age of twenty-one. The HEW guidelines had side-stepped this issue by suggesting that "health experts in the State should be consulted for assistance in establishing periodicity."[110] As a result, the states were much slower to define the periodicity schedule than they had been to define the screening package,[111] and the schedules varied widely enough, as shown in part III, to raise questions about their medical logic.

Finding providers for the screening services caused the states great difficulty. Medicaid itself was not very popular with the medical profession. For example, in New York City fewer than 10 percent of the physicians participated in Medicaid, and state-wide the figure was still reported to be only 40 percent.[112] Physicians explained their unwillingness to see Medicaid patients by claiming that fees were too low and red tape too long. HEW estimated that in 1974 only 51 percent of the physicians and osteopaths in the United States participated in Medicaid. Florida had the lowest participation rate with 30 percent, while West Virginia had the highest with 97 percent.[113] These figures overestimated available medical resources for two reasons: first, a single Medicaid billing would qualify a physician as a participating physician even if he saw no more than one Medicaid eligible person once during a given year; second, health manpower is unevenly distributed in the United States. Many areas, designated formally by HEW as medically under-served, simply lack sufficient medical manpower even if 100 percent were participating in Medicaid. Thus, states faced with a mandate to "provide for" services often found too few providers.

For lack of other resources or for administrative convenience, many states looked toward existing public clinics, the Title V programs run by local or state health departments, to take up the screening program, with referrals to private physicians if further diagnosis and/or treatment were needed. Seventeen states used only health department screening clinics, either using the Title V clinics which already were in place or, in many cases, setting up new clinics or mobile units to cover areas of their states not previously served. Twenty states used a combination of public health departments, private physicians, and hospital outpatient clinics. Thirteen states used no health department clinics, preferring neighborhood clinics, private physicians, and outpatient departments.[114] Problems arose with all the systems. Where private physicians were excluded from screening, they complained, and in one case even sued the state in order to become screening providers.[115] Where private physicians were encouraged to screen children, they often refused, claiming insufficient time, staff, laboratory back-up, or fees.[116]

Nor were relations with the health departments (Title V agencies) necessarily smooth. The health departments wanted to get paid in full for the additional screening which they were undertaking. They saw EPSDT as a way to provide additional financing for their Title V programs which had been held to relatively modest budgetary increases during the 1970s. Thus the contracts were usually worked out through delicate negotiations between health and welfare agencies.

Even if the states succeeded in providing for screening services for most children in one way or another, they still depended on private physicians for diagnosis and treatment. A 1974 survey of eight states noted that none of them could provide all the treatments covered under the state Medicaid plans.[117] Many physicians were apathetic, if not downright hostile to the program.[118] They would have preferred that the EPSDT program work toward the goal of a "medical home" for children and not fragment their care into screening, diagnosis, and treatment in different places.[119] The arrangements with providers which had been a major problem for Medicaid carried over into the EPSDT program, both in terms of finding screening providers and in terms of providing subsequent care.[120] Federal and state administrators tended to emphasize the screening aspects of the program because they assumed that the diagnosis and treatment were readily available under Medicaid. This assumption proved to be wrong, but it was only the existence of EPSDT which uncovered that fact.

To identify children and inform them of the new program were new activities for Medicaid programs. It did no good to identify children if they (or their parents) were not informed of the program. Originally, most states attempted to inform the parents simply by handing them a piece of paper about EPSDT when they first became eligible, or when they came back for recertification for Medicaid. Frequently, they prepared brochures which they handed out or sent out with welfare checks. Some states also used radio and TV bulletins.[121] However, the most effective method to get people to use the services proved to be individual contact, at least by telephone, if not in person.[122] To inform, educate, and then follow up, the states had to allocate staff. Most states allocated the task of informing to the Medicaid agency (usually the welfare department), where it was done by case workers. The follow-up responsibility fell to the health departments in twenty-two states.[123] States tried many different combinations; all were more or less unsatisfactory as they involved at least two agencies and multiple levels of bureaucracy as well as an information system that was virtually non-existent.

Implementation proceeded slowly. The states first off the mark were those which were able to put in place fairly quickly a screening program through the health departments,[124] and those who were under a court order requiring implementation. For example, Michigan, which met both these criteria, early developed a reputation of having one of the better EPSDT programs, in good part because the state's strong health department, when given a contract for screening by the welfare department, was able to put together sufficient services throughout the state.[125] However, having the Title V agency, the health department, as the sole or major contractor for services, did not necessarily assure higher screening levels as the programs progressed.

Nation-wide, between July 1972 and December 1973, 11 percent of the eligible children were reported to have been screened. The numbers ranged from a tenth of 1 percent in Massachusetts to 60 percent in Alabama (table 2). These figures are suspect since they exhibit a certain preference for zero as the final digit in the reported proportions. Twenty-one out of the list of forty-three numbers ended in zero. By chance, one would expect such an occurrence less than one in a thousand times. Such a preference for rounded figures was not difficult to achieve because both the numerator (the number screened) and the denominator (the number eligible) were not reliably reported. By the years 1976 and 1978, the digit preference disappeared, but the reporting problems persisted.

By FY 1976, 16 percent of the eligible children were reported as being screened, with the proportion rising to 20 percent in FY 1978. If one considers the number of children who should have been screened in any one year according to each state's periodicity schedule, the national average was still better, with 28 percent screened in 1978. However, state performances varied from the District of Columbia, with a low of 8 percent, to Wyoming, which miraculously screened 110 percent of those eligible (see table 2). What accounts for these variations? First, the reporting problems mentioned above; second, the different periodicity schedules that are discussed in part III. For the moment, it is sufficient to note that since Wyoming required only three screens for a child between birth and the age of twenty-one, it could more readily be an overachiever than states which required twenty-five screens during the same years. Finally, states were careless in regard to duplicated counts. A review of agencies doing the screening in Connecticut revealed that the actual unduplicated count of children screened was 35 to 40 percent of that reported by the state to the federal government.[126] The duplicate counts existed within each year, and aggregating these counts over several years would then exaggerate the number of different children screened over several years. For example, out of eleven million eligible children, over five million were reported screened between February 1972 and June 1976,[127] but these figures very likely included repeated screenings for the same children. Therefore, the reported figures can only be a rough measure of the number of children who were actually screened.

Another limitation of the data is that if children were screened in doctors' offices, often in conjunction with other care, and if the doctors charged for their services with a Medicaid billing form, the

Table 2 Children eligible for and screened by the EPSDT program, by state, 1973, 1976, 1978

State	Percentage of Eligible Children Screened Under EPSDT Program			Children Screened as a Percentage of Children Who Should Have Been Screened According to State's Periodicity Schedule, FY 1978	Number of Eligible Children, 1978[a]
	July 1972 to Dec. 1973	FY 1976	FY 1978		
Total[b]	11%	16%	20%	28%	10,285,000
Alabama	60	24	27	85	178,000
Alaska	20	34	53	66	10,000
Arizona	No Medicaid Program				
Arkansas	21	23	27	55	96,000
California	0.9	2	11	13	1,172,000
Colorado	14	49	41	50	88,000
Connecticut	8.0	26	27	36	137,000
Delaware	23	30	9	22	27,000
D.C.	3.0	6.0	4	8	103,000
Florida	30	42	32	57	215,000
Georgia	6.0	38	40	82	194,000
Hawaii	20	14	19	31	44,000
Idaho	NA[c]	41	78	89	17,000
Illinois	NA	7	15	22	736,000
Indiana	10	NA	41	59	160,000
Iowa	40	32	28	28	78,000
Kansas	10	20	10	10	109,000
Kentucky	6.0	18	14	14	226,000
Louisiana	30	19	25	45	189,000
Maine	10	17	22	31	62,000
Maryland	5.0	4	10	19	234,000
Massachusetts	0.1	5	34	27	380,000
Michigan	22	18	16	42	653,000
Minnesota	10	6	12	22	136,000
Mississippi	40	31	34	104	208,000
Missouri	20	13	14	14	229,000
Montana	20	10	12	12	13,000
Nebraska	20	32	28	28	37,000
Nevada	30	35	39	65	10,000
New Hampshire	NA	11	19	29	24,000
New Jersey	1.0	10	9	14	464,000
New Mexico	4.0	26	19	32	49,000
New York	40	12	12	18	1,118,000
North Carolina	NA	25	38	30	181,000
North Dakota	50	6.0	22	48	13,000
Ohio	NA	14	10	35	447,000
Oklahoma	40	16	13	13	89,000
Oregon	2.0	34	35	49	99,000
Pennsylvania	NA	24	30	39	614,000

Table 2 (continued)

State	Percentage of Eligible Children Screened Under EPSDT Program			Children Screened as a Percentage of Children Who Should Have Been Screened According to State's Periodicity Schedule, FY 1978	Number of Eligible Children, 1978[a]
	July 1972 to Dec. 1973	FY 1976	FY 1978		
Total[b]	11%	16%	20%	28%	10,285,000
Rhode Island	6.0	9.0	29	59	50,000
South Carolina	50	21	20	61	125,000
South Dakota	1.0	11	27	38	17,000
Tennessee	24	38	29	64	190,000
Texas	12	32	30	60	333,000
Utah	NA	20	15	27	32,000
Vermont	6.0	21	48	73	23,000
Virginia	30	20	20	20	169,000
Washington	5.0	23	34	29	130,000
West Virginia	20	27	32	39	67,000
Wisconsin	3.0	6.0	7.0	10	272,000
Wyoming	8.0	28	18	110	6,000

Sources:

1973: Anne-Marie Foltz, *EPSDT: Lessons for National Health Insurance for Children*, HRPX006848 (Springfield, Va.: National Technical Information Service, 1975), table 4.

1976: U.S., Department of Health, Education, and Welfare, *Data on the Medicaid Program: Eligibility, Services, Expenditures: Fiscal Years 1966–77*, Health Care Financing Administration, Institute for Medicaid Management, 1977, table 26.

1978: U.S., Department of Health, Education, and Welfare, *Data on the Medicaid Program: Eligibility/Services/Expenditures, 1979 Edition (Revised)*, Health Care Financing Administration, Medicare/Medicaid Institute, 1979, table 26, pp. 52–53; U.S., Department of Health, Education, and Welfare, "Comparison of EPSDT Program Costs for Present and Mandated Periodicity Schedules," Office of Child Health, Health Care Financing Administration, 7 December 1978 (unpublished), table 1. See also Anne-Marie Foltz, "The Politics of Prevention: Child Health under Medicaid" (Ph.D. Dissertation, Yale University, 1980), pp. 343–344.

Note: All figures are those reported by the states and were not verified by the federal government. The percentage screened is dependent on the number of children enumerated as eligible. Particularly in the early days of the program, this was at best an estimate.

[a]"Annualized" number derived by multiplying state monthly figures by 1.2 to account for "off and on" factor.

[b]Puerto Rico, Guam, Virgin Islands, Samoa and Trust Territories excluded.

[c]Figures not available.

children's visits were not reported as screens. Moreover, incomplete screens were counted as screens, as is illustrated by the following questioning of a state EPSDT coordinator by a welfare rights lawyer:

Q. Is Mr. Sassarossi correct in saying that a physician can use the Medicaid reimbursement for purposes of EPSDT?
A. Yes.
Q. Will use of this be recorded as EPSDT screen for statistical purposes?
A. No.
Q. So, the physician will be paid for services performed, but not counted for EPSDT?
A. Yes.
. . .
Q. Does the incomplete billing form count as a screen in the statistics of the number of children screened?
A. Yes.
Q. So that if a physician, let's say, leaves out vision and hearing and hemoglobin, it will be counted as an EPSDT screen?
A. Yes.[128]

Massachusetts, for example, claimed that its doctors were seeing most children, but these visits were not recorded as EPSDT screens and could not be verified.[129]

To evaluate the EPSDT program only in terms of the number of children screened is misleading. HEW used screening activity as the criterion to monitor state compliance, and states responded accordingly. However, the purpose of the program was to bring needy children to care; this included screening, diagnosis, and treatment when appropriate. Screening by itself saves no lives.

It proved difficult, however, to assess a state's performance by measures other than screening. Even states with more sophisticated information systems were unable to document the number of children referred from screening who actually received follow-up care.[130] Thus, the only available information could come either from an overview of the screening and follow-up effort or from special evaluation studies which had access to such data for particular sites.

For the first type of information, two officials of the Office of Child Health in the Medical Services Administration were asked to identify those states which they believed, from reports of the regional offices and from the statistics filed, were making a serious effort to implement EPSDT and those states which were making

little effort. Two assumptions were made: that the effort of informing and screening children and providing follow-up care would
increase the expenditures for children and the number of child
recipients; and that increases in the child effort would outstrip
those increases for adults for whom no new programs were
implemented.

The changes in expenditures and recipients in 1972 and 1976
were compared for children and adults in three "strong" states
and two "weak" states. The years 1972 to 1976 saw a rise in overall
Medicaid expenditures and in recipients throughout the country.
However, states with "strong" EPSDT programs, such as Michigan
and South Carolina, had twice the increases in expenditures for
children during that period than they had for adults, and Michigan had also greater increases in child recipients than it had for
adults (table 3). Texas's increases in expenditures for children
barely kept pace with increases for adults, but its number of child
recipients increased notably compared to adults. This is not surprising since the EPSDT program required reaching children in

Table 3 EPSDT and Medicaid services in selected states

	"Strong" EPSDT Programs			"Weak" EPSDT Programs	
	Michigan	Texas	South Carolina	California	Indiana
EPSDT screening expenditures as a percentage of total Medicaid expenditures, 1976	0.6	0.1	0.4	0.05	0.8
Percent change in adult Medicaid expenditures, 1972–1976	112.6	216.8	207.8	76.2	92.2
Percent change in children's Medicaid expenditures, 1972–1976	215.5	189.1	400.3	29.6	4.7
Percent change in adult Medicaid recipients, 1972–1976	60.9	6.8	199.8	–22.2	10.7
Percent change in child Medicaid recipients, 1972–1976	112.6	77.2	192.7	–18.0	10.0

Source: U.S., Department of Health, Education, and Welfare, National Center for
Social Statistics, unpublished data.

areas where medical care had previously been very limited. The two "weak" states, California and Indiana, showed much less investment in child health. The increases in expenditures for children did not keep pace with those for adults, while the changes in numbers of child recipients mirrored those of adults.

Since screening expenditures were usually less than 1 percent of the Medicaid budget (table 3), these procedures themselves would not greatly influence budgets. However, since EPSDT involved screening and treatment, one would expect expenditures to rise as children who needed care were brought into the system. Of course, this assumes that there were children out there who needed care who were not getting it until EPSDT came along, but this fact has been sufficiently well documented to allow such gross comparisons as those in table 3.

How many children are brought into any system of health care is more difficult to assess. A number of evaluations have attempted to ascertain whether sufficient needy children were reached in the EPSDT program, whether those needing follow-up care received it, and whether children received timely rescreens. The studies document some improvement in child health services, but also document much inadequacy in the program. Moreover, it is difficult to generalize from these studies: they are usually from specific sites, and they all suffer from methodological problems. The EPSDT program became a methodological tar baby. Whoever tried to evaluate the program seemed to get stuck on the methods. In part this was due to the complexity of the program, in part it was due to the difficulty of getting reliable data, and in part it was due to the researchers themselves. Many studies were undertaken by advocates or governmental critics of the program; others were under contract to federal agencies (which gave them a particular perspective). Advocates were often as critical of the program's operations as other groups.[131]

The proportion of children referred for follow-up diagnosis and treatment was used as one measure of the efficacy of the EPSDT program. [132] The federal government required collection of such information, and therefore most evaluations used it as well because it was readily available. Nation-wide, the proportion of children reported as referred with at least one condition was just under 50 percent throughout the program's first six years.[133] The range, however, was 4 percent for Vermont to 92 percent for Mississippi.[134] These variations were corroborated by other studies.

Michigan reported 62 percent,[135] while Minnesota had only 30 percent referred.[136] Among the four of five counties studied by the Children's Defense Fund, the proportion referred ranged from 18.8 percent in Florence County, South Carolina, to 94.5 percent in Oktibbeha County, Mississippi.[137]

What accounts for these variations in referral patterns? Can it be that nearly all children in Mississippi had conditions which needed to be treated and nearly none did in Vermont? There are several explanations. First, children would be less likely to be referred if they were screened at a place which offered treatment immediately (and this type of self-referral would not be noted as a referral in the reports). Second, some states would not allow an EPSDT-eligible child to receive mandated dental, vision, or hearing services unless the child were referred from a screening clinic. Since almost all children needed dental services, such states' referral figures would therefore be considerably higher than those of other states. Variations in referral rates also stemmed from different criteria for referrable conditions. It is also possible that screening clinics were less likely to refer a child for a minor condition if they knew that providers of diagnosis and treatment would be hard to find.[138] The quality of the screen is also an important factor: a sloppy job of screening can leave many conditions undetected. Finally, there remains the uncertainty of ascertaining what the true need for treatment was among eligible children. A high yield could show that screening was very effective in finding untreated health problems, or that there were many untreated problems in the community for the screeners to find, or simply that the screeners were overzealous in their work and detecting disease that was not there. Presently available data give no resolution of these issues, and suggest that the proportion of referrals is an inadequate way of evaluating the EPSDT program.

The two states, Connecticut and Texas, which served as cases for the present study illustrate divergent referral patterns and some possible interpretations. Connecticut in fiscal year 1976 referred 44.4 percent of all children screened.[139] The referral rate was lower for those under six years old (35 percent) than for older children (55.8 percent). This resulted because Connecticut's periodicity schedules recommended more repeat screenings for younger children and because these repeat screenings were not distinguished by Connecticut in its reporting. Therefore, younger children, because they were likely to be seen more frequently, were less likely at any particular visit to have conditions requiring referrals.

Texas referred only 28.4 percent of children.[140] However, Texas clinics, unlike providers in Connecticut, did not have to refer children for dental services, because all children were automatically included in a separate dental program. Texas children who were screened more than once during 1973 to 1977 would occasionally be referred again for the same condition for which they had been referred on a previous screening visit. This occurred for 6 percent of urban children and 7 percent of rural children, and may have reflected the difficulty of finding adequate providers for treatment.

A better method to evaluate the program's effectiveness would be to see how great a proportion of children identified as having problems received timely and appropriate care. Alas, most states did not and could not collect such data; only limited evaluation studies of specific sites are available. The House Subcommittee on Oversight and Investigations reported that in nine states, 60 percent of children needing medical treatment received it, but failed to document how these data were collected.[141] Another study, with methodological problems of its own, reported 78 percent of children needing care received it.[142] The Children's Defense Fund reported a follow-up of 84 percent in a New Jersey county, 50 percent in a Michigan county, 46 percent in a Mississippi county, and 39 percent in a South Carolina county.[143] In another study, the efficacy of follow-up seemed to be improved in an experimental program in which children were followed by special case monitors who facilitated their screening and treatment. Among the experimental group, 70.1 percent of problems were resolved, while among a control group, only 37.8 percent of the problems were resolved.[144]

All in all, there remains little solid information on the extent of follow-up after screening. If it proved difficult to find clinics or persons to provide screening services, it was an even greater chore to find physicians willing to perform the necessary and concomitant diagnosis and treatment. What sparse data there are indicate that anywhere from 30 to 60 percent of children did not receive the treatment which should have followed from these screenings, if the screening findings themselves were valid.

In summary, although it is difficult to generalize about a program which was different in forty-nine states, certain points can nevertheless be made about services under EPSDT. First, preventive services had not as a rule been available to Medicaid-eligible children before Medicaid. In 1978, after five years of operation, the EPSDT program nation-wide managed to screen annually 28 percent of those who should have received such services. However, a modest proportion of this figure represents repeat screenings of the same children. Moreover, state service patterns varied widely. State Medicaid agencies, undertaking tasks new for them, set standards for care including which screening tests should be performed and what the periodicity schedules should be, resulting in considerable variation among the states. State Medicaid agencies had severe problems getting sufficient providers for screening and for treatment. Contrary to expectations, Title V agencies (the health departments) in most states did not provide screening or treatment services for most children. Private physicians were also reluctant to participate. Nevertheless, the states with the higher rates of screening tended to be those which involved health departments. States also used other providers such as outpatient departments of hospitals, neighborhood health centers, and mobile units. Overall, the implementation of the program was very slow.

Evaluation of program services must include the question of whether children referred needed referral and, if so, if they got appropriate treatment. Depending on the state, at least 40 to 70 percent of children screened who needed care did receive that care. Present studies cannot provide any more reliable figures, because the "need" for services has not been defined. This study of implementation therefore cannot provide any better data even in the two states surveyed because the states have not collected reliable data.

Costs

During the 1970s, federal and state expenditures for Medicaid services grew steadily. From $6.5 billion in 1971, they rose to $19.6 billion in 1979.[145] Most of the increase could be attributed to the rise in hospital and nursing home costs, but some could also be attributed to the expansion of services and eligibility. By 1975, however, states were turning to ways of cutting costs by cutting benefits,[146] or by cutting back the number of eligible persons. California, for example, minimized cost increases by changing its eligibility standards and removing the medically needy from coverage. (See table 3 for the effect of these changes.) States would have cut back more than they did if they had not faced the constant threat of suits from welfare rights lawyers.

Most Medicaid costs, particularly those of hospitalization, seemed uncontrollable. It is therefore no wonder that the states did not enthusiastically pursue the EPSDT program. State welfare directors were having a difficult enough time defending their massive welfare and Medicaid budgets before skeptical state legislators without having to add even a small amount for a special child health program. To obtain providers of services, welfare directors often had to contract with health departments, the Title V agencies. However, these agencies, having been on short funds for most of their existence, were not inclined to provide services unless they were adequately compensated. In some states, such as Connecticut, getting compensation for the health agency proved impossible because whatever funds the welfare agency paid would go into the state's general fund and not be allocated to the health department. Thus, there were no incentives to cooperate because of the state's method of budgeting and financing. States soon found themselves trapped in complex negotiations for payment, case finding, case monitoring, and services, with a patchwork of public and private providers of care.

In 1971, when the Office of Management and Budget had finally approved regulations for the EPSDT program, the estimated annual cost was $25 million. By 1975, state and federal screening expenditures alone had risen to $34 million; three years later they were still going up to $48 million.[147] These figures excluded many other costs, such as administration, information systems, case finding, case monitoring, and the costs of additional treatment for children found to need care. Administrative costs and information systems for EPSDT were always a part of overall Medicaid administrative costs, but because administrative resources were never heavily applied to the program, they probably remained low. More important, they proved virtually impossible to identify.[148] States, at first, did not link Medicaid treatment with EPSDT screening data, so it proved impossible to estimate state-wide costs of treatment following from screening. Thus, the only available data on these costs come from special studies or demonstration projects which kept separate information on the local costs of case finding, case monitoring, and treatment. Such data exclude the state-wide administrative and information costs mentioned above.

Costs for treatment services did increase slightly for children screened.[149] However, no study followed the children for more than one year after screening. It is hard to evaluate the long-term effects of the screening program on Medicaid costs in such a short time span since health needs fluctuate widely at different ages; the randomness of illnesses is probably a much stronger explanatory factor for fluctuations in treatment costs.

As for the costs of case finding, monitoring, and follow-up for children in certain demonstration projects, the Dallas demonstration project ran up costs of $100.10 per child screened.[150] This included the screening costs and dental services as well, but not other treatment. If one were to overcome one's methodological misgivings and extrapolate this figure, and if the country were to have screened in 1978 all seven million children who were eligible according to the states' periodicity schedules, the cost of the program that year would have been $700 million. Of course, this is only speculation; the Dallas estimates may have been high; the children required by state periodicity schedules to be screened was certainly higher than medically necessary. Nevertheless, EPSDT was evidently a program which in implementation would cost a great deal more than the $25 million OMB had acknowledged back in 1971.

One must keep in mind that when President Johnson submitted the original EPSDT legislation to Congress, he had suggested that over $100 million additional be allocated to Medicaid for the purposes of this program. The federal Medicaid budget did increase that year and in following years, but the additional funds did not, except in small measure, go for the EPSDT program. The reason was that ultimately it was the states that decided how much to spend on EPSDT. They spent relatively little and thereby managed to keep the costs relatively low.

As people grew increasingly concerned with the cost of the public programs, critics charged the EPSDT program with being cost-increasing and not cost-effective. These two statements should be separated: the program certainly was, and should be, cost-increasing since it was designed to provide screening (preventive) services to children who had hitherto received none. The services also included treatment, particularly for vision, hearing, and dental care. Only the most naive individual could expect this mandate to reduce Medicaid costs, at least in the short run. That such services would be cost-effective, that they would save unnecessary crippling and concomitant costs for thousands of children, was a firmly held but untested assumption of the framers of the legislation. This assumption could have been tested once the program was in place, but none of the evaluations did so successfully. Unable to prove its effectiveness, the program stood defenseless against critics reluctant to spend more money on the "unworthy" poor.

Incrementalism at Work

The problems which were built into the original EPSDT legislation were not resolved during its first eleven years. Subsequent congressional and HEW neglect compounded them. The Title V agencies could not fulfill the vision of the legislation's framers and provide the EPSDT program with a structure. Title V had limited itself to caring for those not otherwise cared for—a series of stop-gap measures that defined coverage by present demand. EPSDT increased the demand for services, which overwhelmed many health departments. The Title V programs had also, except for their projects, limited themselves to screening. Therefore, those states which used Title V agencies fragmented and dissociated screening from treatment.

The states viewed EPSDT as a federal program. The states themselves had little incentive to implement it, because it would increase their Medicaid costs. The federal matching percentages were not sufficient to make states want to spend their own money on a program that states themselves were not interested in. Fortunately, some were.

EPSDT confronted the state Medicaid agencies with an entirely new type of program. Previously, they had been content with paying bills as filed to them and with monitoring fraud and abuse. The federal government thrust the responsibility upon them to make contracts with providers of care, to identify eligible children, to inform them of the services available, and to monitor appropriate follow-up; this was beyond the scope and interests of most Medicaid agencies. Both the federal and state governments underestimated the complexity of the administrative task. Almost all the states had insufficient information systems to cope with a monitoring program, and the agencies were permanently short-staffed. Moreover, some of the decisions they had to make, such as establishing the periodicity schedules for screening, were well beyond the talents of most of the staffs. Finally, they had to find providers to serve the Medicaid children, a formidable task for many states with limited health resources.

Despite all these problems, the EPSDT program delivered screening services to large numbers of children who had previously not received preventive care. Many of these children were given needed follow-up care, even if that care was sometimes inadequate.

EPSDT is a classic case of incremental policy-making. Beyond the initial idea that something should be done to screen children and prevent potentially crippling disease lay no comprehensive vision of what EPSDT should be. It "just grow'd" in response to political, bureaucratic, and administrative forces inherent in America's complex federal system. The incrementalism was itself not a matter of chance. It was part of the EPSDT framers' strategy to build a broad program with as little disruption of existing structures as possible. The advantage of such an incremental approach is that it minimizes opposition because it threatens no structures. The disadvantage is that it creates no major structure with a stake in preserving the program. As we shall see, incrementalism does not necessarily run only one way. EPSDT, lacking strong political and bureaucratic support, remained vulnerable to decrementalism.

II | *Institutional Constraints*

For forms of government let fools contest;
Whate'er is best administer'd is best.
Alexander Pope, *Essays on Man*

Federal-State Relations

Federal-state relations have long perplexed thoughtful observers. Sundquist and Davis found the key issue to be the degree of bureaucratic and programmatic coordination between the two levels of government.[1] Sanford, however, as a former state governor, saw the federal government as an overwhelming presence which needed to be controlled and coordinated.[2] He envisioned American federalism as based increasingly on coercion from Washington. Another view of the American federalist system is "this dreamy monster . . . the most inefficient body for spending money on non-specific and non-measured objectives that could be conceived."[3] This vision presents the federal system as an undisciplined marketplace devoid of central coordination.

The federal government has a limited number of ways to carry out its policies in the states and localities. In matters of health and welfare, it has assumed it can buy the cooperation of the states primarily by offering to pay part of a state's share for a given program. Some careful observers have noted that such federal grant programs do influence state programs and policies, at least indirectly.[4] However, others have argued that grants most often just permit the states to do what they would have done anyway.[5]

The EPSDT program is a case where cooperation between federal and state agencies was at a minimum. Washington required all states with a Medicaid program to undertake EPSDT. Under federal-state agreements, the federal government reimbursed states for part of their expenses for the program. However, the states' agreement to accept federal funds did not, as it turned out, mean they complied with federal regulations. Noncompliance occurred even though Congress had supplemented the federal agency's ability to obtain cooperation through financial inducement by voting it powers to exact penalties from states who remained recalcitrant. To understand why Washington had so little influence over state policy despite the usual compliance mechanisms and the additional penalty mandated by Congress, one must review how the federal government used penalties to garner state cooperation.

Grants and Compliance

The federal government has used three types of grants in order to stimulate states to inaugurate or expand programs. General revenue sharing grants, first introduced by Congress in 1972, are distributed by formula with few or no limits on the purposes for which they may be used. Block grants, also distributed by formula, are for broad general purposes such as the comprehensive health planning grants of 1966 or the Community Development Act of 1974, both of which consolidated existing grant programs while broadening the state and locality's mandate. Both such grants provide greater flexibility for the states and require relatively little federal monitoring.

Categorical grants which allocate funds for specific purposes have been the most common and have involved greater dollar amounts.[6] Categorical grants take three forms: formula grants give each state a certain sum based on a formula which takes account of population or income distribution; project grants require states and localities to compete for funds; and open-ended reimbursement grants reimburse states a fixed percentage of their expenses for a categorical program. Under reimbursement grants the federal matching percentages are those that are assumed to provide incentives for state spending. Thus, poorer states would be encouraged to participate because the federal government would offer to pay a higher percentage of their costs than it would for wealthier states. That, at least, is the theory.

Medicaid was a categorical open-ended grant which reimbursed states from 50 to 83 percent of their expenses for medical assistance, depending upon the per capita income of the state. The states were free to participate or not to participate in the program. The incentive for a state was the federal matching percentage; the disincentive was the additional cost to state taxpayers of an expanded welfare program. One state, Arizona, continued to refuse to participate all through the 1970s.[7]

To receive federal funds, states had to draft a state plan acceptable to the federal government, and then abide by that plan. The compliance procedures, originally laid down for the Public Assistance grants and later applied to Medicaid, proved to be weak instruments for enforcing federal laws. The main tool of compliance was to withhold funds, but this tool was unwieldy. Administrative procedures required first negotiations between the federal agency and the noncompliant state. Only if these (often lengthy) negotiations failed could the issue go to a public hearing. After the public hearing, more negotiations could ensue. Moreover, the federal guidelines noted, "in practice, hearings have been a last resort."[8] The history of Public Assistance reveals few cases of public hearings and no cases of total funds actually being withheld. The most expeditious way of circumventing federal mandates was to have the mandate itself changed by Congress, something Indiana succeeded in doing in 1951 after it was brought to a public hearing for noncompliance.[9]

The weakness of the compliance procedures lay in part in the administrative process and in part in the fact that to withdraw state funds would penalize not the state, but the poor and needy people which the federal program was designed to serve. Thus, federal reluctance to use what little power it had is not surprising.

In Medicaid, as with Public Assistance, funds were never withheld completely, despite more than twenty-three hundred incidents of state noncompliance with federal regulations during the program's first ten years.[10] The federal government never moved to compliance procedures under Medicaid because officials feared that the subsequent hearings could keep them tied up in the courts for years and years.[11] They did have "strong conversations" with the states,[12] and they did disallow for certain types of expenditures when negotiating payments for future quarters. However, these amounts were relatively small.[13]

Using compliance procedures for EPSDT proved no more effective than for Medicaid as a whole. Beginning in 1972, HEW had added EPSDT requirements to the list of compliance issues. However, nine of the fifteen states that were found in compliance with EPSDT in the first compliance review had submitted no concrete evidence to show they had any sort of program actually in operation.[14] The General Accounting Office found that compliance failures in seven states had been noted in several quarterly reports from the regional offices, but that HEW had held no formal compliance hearings.[15]

The EPSDT Penalty

Since available compliance procedures had proved worthless, it is not surprising that the idea of a penalty should arise. Such a penalty would apply to only a small part of state funds; hence, it was theorized, it would not create such a hardship on the recipients of services or on the states.

This kind of thinking lay behind the congressional decision in 1972 to apply a 1 percent penalty to AFDC funds for states which failed to comply with EPSDT. This decision itself had occurred in a last minute reversal of policy: while the House of Representatives had contemplated eliminating EPSDT altogether, the Senate, attempting to strengthen it, had voted a 2 percent penalty for failure to implement the program. The Conference Report compromise reduced this to 1 percent.[16] The penalty was to be applied to the federal share of AFDC funds of any state in any quarter if it failed to

(1) inform all families in the State receiving aid to families with dependent children . . . of the availability of child health screening services [under Medicaid]. . . .
(2) provide or arrange for the provision of such screening services in all cases where they are requested, or
(3) arrange for (directly or through referral to appropriate agencies, organizations, or individuals) corrective treatment the need for which is disclosed by such child health screening services.[17]

The law was to take effect in July 1974. Congress had thus given HEW an enforcement tool. The EPSDT program was now to become a battleground to test federal strength against the states. As Steiner noted, the program had "become an enforcement challenge, a test of relative determination, not a cooperative effort to accomplish an agreed objective."[18] Whether HEW might have been able to use its new enforcement tool had it been interested is an unanswerable question, because HEW's policy toward EPSDT between 1972 and the end of the decade remained uncertain.

Just as with the original EPSDT legislation, as long as there were no regulations, there would be no implementation of the penalty. Only after much unfavorable publicity did HEW draft and publish regulations, which appeared on 2 August 1974, one month after the law was to take effect.[19]

Although enforcement could now begin, it proved to be slow and erratic. The regional offices were asked to file reports on states for the first quarter of fiscal 1975 (July through September 1974). By November, most of the reports were duly filed. Eight months later, on 2 June 1975, the Secretary of HEW finally cited seven states for noncompliance during the first reporting period. The states in question—Hawaii, Indiana, Minnesota, Montana, New

Mexico, North Dakota, and Pennsylvania—had been warned of what was coming. By the end of the year, two more states, California and New York, had been added to the penalty list. By the end of 1976, Pennsylvania, Hawaii, California, New Mexico, Indiana, and New York had been cited also for the second quarter of 1975. All the states protested and asked for reconsideration. To emphasize their protest, some states, such as Hawaii, also had their congressional delegations call on the Secretary of HEW. The states stood to lose collectively a total of only $12.3 million in AFDC funds if the decision after reconsideration were unfavorable. However, by mid-1977, HEW had made no decision. In the interim, many people, both in and out of HEW, had pointed out that the regulations might be unenforceable.

Penalty reports continued to be filed for the last two quarters of fiscal 1975 and for fiscal 1976, but no new penalties were announced. For these later rounds of penalty monitoring, states which had been found in compliance the previous quarter were monitored only every other quarter. Thus Indiana could be found to be "in compliance" by the regional office, while observers within the state were reporting serious deficiencies.[20] By early 1977, monitoring of the penalty regulations had essentially stopped, although the states were not formally told until March 1978.

Uncertainty about the regulations had caused HEW to publish proposed revised regulations in August 1975.[21] These had elicited much comment—with most of that from the states being unfavorable—with the result that rather than publish final regulations, HEW published another set of proposed regulations in September 1977.[22] This set, too, received much comment, again unfavorable from the states, but with strong support from children's advocacy groups and legal aid organizations. After these latter groups had mobilized sufficient concern and publicity, final regulations were published in May 1979, with an effective date of October of that same year.[23] During the following six months HEW undertook a trial monitoring of the states and scheduled penalty monitoring under the 1979 regulations to begin on 1 July 1980, eight years after the law was enacted.

Reasons for the Penalty's Failure

Why had eight years elapsed from passage of the penalty provision without a single penalty being levied against the states, when all the evidence pointed to their failure to carry out the program? The federal government had won a number of battles to maintain the penalty but seemed to have lost the war. States could continue to hope that it would just be a matter of time until HEW or its 1980 successor, the Department of Health and Human Services (HHS), withdrew its penalizing troops from the field. There are five possible explanations for HEW's inability to use the penalty effectively.

First, the regulations as first published in 1974, then revised in 1975 and 1977, were as ambiguous as the law they were designed to enforce. As a later HEW memo noted:

The lack of clear and reasonable EPSDT penalty regulations has been a significant barrier to effective implementation of the program. Penalty regulations issued in 1974 could not be administered because they did not contain specific requirements against which compliance could be tested.[24]

They required states to inform children, but did not specify what was meant by informing; they specified that states had to provide screening or care within a certain period of time, if requested,[25] but until 1979 did not specify what documentation the state had to collect to show its compliance with requests. Screening was required if requested, but only in the 1977 proposed regulations did HEW first specify what procedures constituted a complete screen.

The ambiguity on required screening procedures was due in no small part, as we shall see in part III, to the scientific controversy surrounding screening. For example, in 1975 the Director of Public Information of the American Academy of Pediatrics in Wisconsin charged that that state's screening procedures "remain an unproved method of disease finding and have been strongly condemned by this Society."[26]

As the regulations evolved, the most perplexing question was whether states should be evaluated by documented effort or by documented outcome. States complained that the early forms of the regulations were too specific on every item of process which the states had to follow to notify children and their parents of the program.[27] One Minnesota county administrator noted that "it is conceivable that the proposed documentation requirements could be fulfilled without successfully placing one child in the screening program."[28]

As a result, the regulations of 1979 required less detailed process and substituted specific outcome goals such as that at least 95 percent of a sample of cases reviewed by HEW must be documented to have met the requirements for informing.[29] Nevertheless, considerable ambiguity remained, because the procedures for informing, screening, and providing treatment did not easily lend themselves to codification. This was as much due to the uncertainty of screening as a policy as to anything inherent in federal-state relations.

The 1979 regulations, by substituting documented performance criteria for process criteria, removed some of the ambiguity from the penalty regulations, but created other dismaying problems. Under the new regulations states could incur the penalty even where HEW found only *one* instance of documented noncompliance in its review. Thus, the attempt at clarification and removal of ambiguity confronted HEW administrators with the possibility that fiscal penalties as a cure for state recalcitrance might prove worse than the disease.

This concern for the effectiveness of the penalty constituted the *second* reason for non-enforcement. To many people in HEW and even to some child advocates, the idea of fiscal penalties was philosophically repugnant because withdrawing funds tended not to penalize the states directly, but rather the clients whom the programs were designed to serve. Early in 1975, the director of the Medicaid program had said:

Using the penalty is a double edged sword. The people who get hurt under it are most times the program recipients. We would rather encourage the states through a positive incentive.[30]

This message could not have been clearer when Secretary of HEW F. David Matthews announced $2 million in penalties for New York, and then added:

I have publicly stated my concern about the net effectiveness of this type of sanction since the burden falls on the intended beneficiaries, and since, in this case, it may make matters worse rather than leading to improvements.[31]

These are strong and surprising words for an official responsible for enforcing federal law. The following January, just before he and the Republican administration left office, Matthews refused to sign the revised regulation which had been on his desk for some time and advised his successor, Joseph Califano, to do likewise.

The questions raised about the appropriateness of the application of the penalty caused concern. If Congress had wanted to avoid penalizing the intended beneficiaries of policy, it could have directed that the penalty be applied to state administrative funds. However, because all state funds are fungible this might have worked no better. It would not matter against which state funds penalties were levied since states would always be likely to pass on some of that deficit to their clients.

Nevertheless, there was a particular administrative illogicality to the penalty requirement by the time it was applied. The Medicaid program would incur the penalty, but AFDC would lose the money. In states where these two programs were functionally separate, the penalty made little sense, as California, Texas, and Tennessee protested. This discrepancy became more evident in 1977 when HEW was reorganized and Medicaid, which had been with AFDC in the Social and Rehabilitation Service, was moved into the Health Care Financing Administration (HCFA). As a result, penalties became more and more unpopular with HEW officials, and their application became more and more implausible.

The *third* reason stemmed from the fact that the central HEW office did not control the ten regional offices which actually carried out penalty reviews. Since central HEW was dependent on the latter for information, it often did not know what was going on in the states. Penalty reviews were found to be of "uneven accuracy and thoroughness."[32] Their quality varied

according to how much support EPSDT has from the Administrator of the regional office, the number of staff who work on EPSDT, the staff's interest in EPSDT and their competence in administration and enforcement, and the extent to which the regional office staff are willing to make objective judgments of states' performance, independent of pressures from interest groups and officials in the states.[33]

In addition, there was often "insufficient documentation to indicate the basis upon which . . . conclusions were drawn."[34] Not infrequently states would get different readings from the regional and central offices. For example, in early 1977, the Boston Regional Director wrote Connecticut that if the state did not acquire staff to inform children about EPSDT services, the Boston Regional Office would apply the penalty. However, when Connecticut's Senator Ribicoff, alerted by distressed state officials, took up the matter in Washington, he was assured by HCFA officials that there would be no penalties.[35]

Finally, some states with seemingly similar implementation

problems were cited for penalties and others were not, depending upon which regional office did the monitoring. Inconstancy, then, proved to be the hallmark of the first round of penalty monitoring. The autonomy of the regional offices decreased the effectiveness of the penalty process and made it easier in some regions for states to resist.

This state resistance was the *fourth* reason for HEW's inability to use the penalty effectively. Resistance took several forms: pressure of congressmen on HEW; requests for reconsideration of the penalties; objections to the proposed penalty regulations duly filed during the comment period; and, finally, passive resistance, simply not carrying out programs. HEW received over one hundred comments, most of them negative, for both the 1975 and 1977 proposed regulations. More than half the states wrote; often both health and welfare agencies filed critiques. The Governor of Connecticut felt that "implementation of these proposed regulation changes would impose unnecessary hardships on a program already overburdened with administrative problems."[36] Even Michigan, which had a relatively effective EPSDT program and was in no danger of being penalized, argued against the financial penalty, preferring financial incentives.[37] Protest to the fiscal sanctions extended to the National Association of Counties.[38] This was not surprising since in most of the United States other than New England the task of implementation fell to the counties, and the costs were often shared with state governments. The opinion of the states could not have been stated more succinctly than by the National Governors' Conference: "Without question, passing on of sanctions in the form of a reduction of services for recipients—such as is the case with the Early and Periodic Screening, Diagnosis, and Treatment Program—should be prohibited."[39] The governors, who preferred carrots to sticks, called for replacing penalty provisions with fiscal incentives.[40] To bureaucratic coordination or administrative coercion, they preferred being bought.

States were most concerned with the amount of paperwork the EPSDT program required, particularly the penalty provisions. The elaborate administrative procedures to assure case finding, follow-up, and documentation were all bound to raise costs. Some states felt that the penalty was adding requirements without extra financing. They seemed to miss the point that all the penalty was doing was enforcing a law already on the books, albeit ignored.

The states were prepared to fight anything which would increase their costs. If they undertook the necessary administrative procedures and documentation, and paid for screening and treating additional children who requested care, their costs would rise rapidly. If they resisted, they would be penalized and their costs would rise. Some states, in desperation, evaluated the costs of both options and concluded that penalties might be cheaper than the program,[41] although HEW insisted that this was not a serious option.[42] State officials during this period were under increasing fiscal constraints within their own states. They could scarcely afford to be seen as losing money to the federal government through negligent administration, even if the amounts were small. They were fighting, they believed, on a matter of principle, regardless of the small sums involved. Thus, they had no choice but to fight the penalties, and HEW's wavering gave them no small encouragement.

The *fifth* reason for HEW's inability to use the penalty is the simultaneous occurrence of three types of activities within HEW and without which affected both the program and HEW administrators.[43] The first two activities, which have already been discussed, were the penalty monitoring and the regulation revisions. Through both of these, HEW received constant feedback from the states about implementation problems and the burden the federal government was imposing by attempting to levy a penalty.

The third activity, congressional revision of the EPSDT program, began in early 1977. Like EPSDT itself, it also began in HEW, from where it moved to Congress. As the new legislation, called CHAP,[44] developed, it became increasingly clear that while it would expand EPSDT, it would also minimize the need for a penalty by substituting financial incentives.

Each of these three activities affected the others. As a result, HEW administrators were constantly looking over their shoulders trying to anticipate what would happen next, and whether they should do anything at all about them. (See appendix 1 for the sequence of these three activities.)

Since the new legislation was a major factor in the lack of penalty enforcement, let us examine it in more detail. In the fall of 1976, an economist from Brookings, Karen Davis, who had already published several studies on Medicaid and child health, was approached by the Children's Defense Fund for assistance in revising the EPSDT law to make more children eligible for care and make it more workable administratively. When, under the new Democratic administration in January 1977, Davis became Deputy Assistant Secretary for Planning and Evaluation for Health in HEW, she began circulating within HEW drafts of revisions of EPSDT. The original proposals called for an additional outlay of a modest $250 million to increase the number of children eligible for the program and to provide incentives to the states by raising the matching rate for EPSDT to a maximum of 90 percent.

Newly inaugurated, President Jimmy Carter was greatly interested in a major child health initiative and announced that such a program would be forthcoming. However, when confronted by the cost and the prospect of a 90 percent matching rate, he backed down. He held the program to a maximum of $180 million and a 75 percent matching rate. Carter, as a former governor, was concerned that anything more would make it too easy for the states. Many of those who had worked with the program in HEW were convinced that any rate lower than 90 percent would not encourage state participation.[45] However, the planning went forward on the basis Carter stipulated. The major child health initiative was scaled down. By the time the legislation was sent to Congress it was scarcely noticed, because simultaneously his administration, under the glare of publicity, submitted its cost containment program. CHAP was virtually buried. It was not an auspicious beginning.

The administration bill, sent to Congress on 25 April 1977, called for repeal of the existing penalties after September 1977 and for a new penalty which would be applied to no more than 20 percent of the states' administrative costs.[46] HEW had just announced the states cited for penalties for the second quarter of 1975. The possibility of withdrawal or modification of the sanction gave HEW officials little incentive to pursue the penalty vigorously. However, both the House and Senate delayed action. Not until summer of the following year did a House Committee report out a bill. This one provided for the repeal of the current penalty retroactive to enactment.[47] The retroactive provision would obviate the need for any further penalty monitoring. The accompanying report noted:

The Committee heard considerable testimony on the poor track record of the Department [HEW] in implementing the EPSDT program. We have been extremely concerned by the footdragging on the part of the Department in issuing regulations and in vigorously carrying out the charges of EPSDT.[48]

In anticipation of CHAP's passage, HEW officials had already announced suspension of further penalty reviews. HCFA had also held up publication of final penalty regulations. The move was premature, for in the concluding bustle of the Ninety-Fifth Congress, CHAP, like many other pieces of social legislation, failed to pass. Included in the casualties were Carter's much touted cost containment legislation, health planning, and the creation of a separate Department of Education. The last legislation was to make it through the next Congress. CHAP was not as fortunate. Well aware that CHAP might not succeed, the Children's Defense Fund, which had been active in the struggle for CHAP and had earlier published its own study of EPSDT, pressed for the publication of final regulations. The Children's Defense Fund noted that during the three years since publication of the 1975 proposed regulations, "there had been serious confusion on the part of the states regarding program requirements."[49]

In the next Congress, the administration and several congressmen reintroduced CHAP. By the time the House Committee reported it out, not only had the original penalty been eliminated, but the new one, applied to administrative funds, was directly tied to a minimum state performance, a minimum above which most states were then operating. The framers also managed to tie the matching rate to a state's performance. Thus, if CHAP were passed, there would very likely be no need to apply a penalty at all and states would see the federal government's matching share rise if they maintained high performance levels.[50] This shift in enforcement strategy reflected HEW's increasing disenchantment with the penalty, and congressional frustration at inaction over EPSDT.

By the end of the year, the House of Representatives had finally passed CHAP, but an array of last-minute amendments, including several anti-abortion ones, were sufficient to discourage its advocates and raise questions about its ultimate success. By mid-1980, the Senate had still not reported out a bill, and CHAP died when the Ninety-Sixth Congress adjourned without taking action at the end of 1980. The subsequent Republican administration and more conservative Congress of 1981, concerned with balancing the budget, proposed no improvements for EPSDT.

The congressional uncertainty on CHAP reinforced whatever weaknesses HEW had shown in attempting to enforce the penalty. Caught between an ambiguous mandate and pressures to act, HEW could neither take clear action nor do nothing. The multiple and concurrent interactions among Congress, the White House, HEW, and the states may be characteristic of a federalist system, but they also create great uncertainty in policy development.

Limits of Federalism

By 1980, EPSDT was still not being carried out in many states. HEW had still not succeeded in levying any sanctions against the offenders. All but one of the explanations given for HEW's failure to use the penalty provision to enforce EPSDT point to problems in the federal-state structure. The first explanation has more to do with the problem of defining the purposes of a program as diffuse as EPSDT when a clear consensus was lacking as to what should be done. This issue will be explored further in part III. The four other explanations relate directly or indirectly to the federal struc tures and constitute constraints created by the very institutions through which policy and programs must pass.

The idea of fiscal penalties was philosophically inconsistent in a federalist system based upon the assumption that relations between the states and the federal government should be cooperative rather than coercive. Such thinking then inhibited federal officials from taking action where they might. Moreover, the administrative illogic of applying that particular penalty to AFDC funds may have strengthened the philosophical resolve not to institute the penalty.

HEW could not control the regional offices, the layer of bureaucracy which lay between it and the states. The Nixon administration had strengthened the autonomy of these offices in order to increase decentralization and weaken the power of the Washington bureaucracy. However, once this was accomplished, it proved impossible for the central office to monitor either the states or the regional offices' monitoring of the states.

State resistance to the penalty, which arose mainly out of a concern for costs, were as much part of the resistance to implementing EPSDT as a whole as to the particular aspects of the penalty. Even though the $12 million in penalties assessed was miniscule compared to nearly $18 billion of Medicaid expenditures, states would fight about any amount. This state resistance, coupled with the many activities of regulation writing and legislative drafting, increased Washington's propensity to do nothing about the program.

One must not look upon the EPSDT penalty as an isolated case.

Simultaneously, the federal government was dispensing grants in hundreds of categorical programs and overseeing state compliance. One can also imagine that there were trade-offs between state and federal agencies, that the federal government might push compliance on some grants rather than others. Nevertheless, EPSDT was a special case in that Congress had added a penalty procedure to the usual compliance procedures.

The penalty should have worked better than compliance procedures, it was theorized, because the states should have felt less threatened by withdrawal of only 1 percent of AFDC funds than by withdrawal of all funds. That they did not was due in large part to state resistance to any EPSDT program and to the very concept of a penalty, no matter what its size.

The states may have succeeded in resisting the penalty in large part because HEW was in such disarray over EPSDT policy. EPSDT had been launched with much uncertainty and ambiguity. HEW had continued to administer the program uncertainly and ambiguously through two Republican administrations. By the time a Democratic administration took over in 1977, it was expected, at least by child advocates and some civil servants within HEW, that this uncertainty and ambiguity would cease. In fact, it persisted. President Carter was as ambiguous as his predecessors on EPSDT policy, and state resistance was as strong as ever.

What, then, are the lessons of this experience in non-enforcement? First, bureaucratic coordination, in the form of extensive monitoring, reporting, and review procedures, does not produce effective federal-state cooperation. It is possible—though not probable on the evidence of this case—that executive leadership from a president and a secretary willing to expend political capital to coerce and cajole compliance might have permitted bureaucratic coordination to work. Such was not forthcoming. The fumbling of HEW and successive presidents on EPSDT left the states with wide latitude to attack a costly and unwanted program.

The second lesson is that if you want enforcement of federal policy, coercion in the form of sanctions does not work either. The availability of a penalty provision was no better a solution than the cumbersome compliance procedures. Once states were determined not to comply they could do so as easily under one system as another. Small penalties turned out to be no easier to administer than the threat of removing all funds.

Would matching rates higher than the then existing 50 to 83 percent provide any greater incentives? At times, Congress and/or HEW offered the states higher matching rates for particular Medicaid programs. Washington eventually received good compliance when it offered the states a 90 percent matching rate for the development of Medicaid Management Information Systems. However, the 75 percent matching rate available to states for case finding for the EPSDT program did not elicit much response. One problem was the administrative headache for states of calculating the federal contribution for programs having different matching rates. However, the major problem was the incentive: whether the existing matching rates supplied sufficient incentives for the states. It has been argued that if the federal government paid 100 percent, states would have no incentive to be administratively efficient. But lower matching rates of 50 to 83 percent do not seem to have produced high state cooperation with federal policies. It seems that the price for buying state cooperation lies somewhere between 90 and 100 percent, depending on the degree of state apathy or active hostility toward a given program. It may be politic to refer to this relationship as cooperative or to decry it as coercive. The fact is that when the matching rate goes this high, the federal government is simply exercising its economic power in what is a marketplace relationship with the states.

Health and Welfare Ideologies

This chapter investigates the hypothesis that the organizational ideologies of implementing agencies acted as a significant constraint on the EPSDT program's ability to carry out its task. If this were to be the case, we should expect that variations in performance would be associated in regular fashion with the ideology of the type of organization responsible for implementing the program.

The question is particularly relevant because EPSDT straddled two administrative traditions—health and welfare. This is not just an analytic judgment taken in hindsight; at the implementation stage HEW officials repeatedly raised the question of whether EPSDT were basically a health or welfare program. As late as 1977, and again in 1978, the possibility was raised of transferring EPSDT, at least at the federal level, from the Health Care Financing Administration (welfare) to the Public Health Service (health).[51] Officials were motivated less by a philosophical desire for definitional precision than by a pragmatic search for guidance in assigning administrative responsibility to that part of HEW's vast structure most likely to possess the bureaucratic ideology and operating procedures congruent with EPSDT's nature. Participants in these discussions asked what were the actual functions of welfare as opposed to health agencies and whether one were more appropriate than the other for carrying out EPSDT's assigned tasks.

Ideology is the publicly enunciated way a bureaucracy states its goals, values, and beliefs. Organizational goals are usually not highly specific; the decision-making system is a loosely coupled one.[52] In the best sense, bureaucratic ideology is the bureaucracy's assessment of what the public interest is. It can be viewed as an arena of conflict between "social values" and "organizational values" where one type of value is more likely to predominate than another.[53] Organizational values may be important as they may involve maintaining or expanding the agency or emphasizing its own high efficiency.[54] Implicit in the HEW officials' search for definition was the assumption that underlying organizational ideology also constitutes a prime constraint on performance.

Organizational ideology may be understood to embody three

levels of goals on a continuum from the abstract and general to the concrete and specific. The highest level involves generalized social goals usually embodied in highly general statements of purpose: How does an organization conceptualize its task? The next level involves more specific administrative goals of efficiency and organizational maintenance: How does an organization relate its own structures to its task? The third, and most specific, involves service goals which specify the particular services an agency is expected to render to the public: How does it translate the more general goals into specific programmatic actions?

The method chosen in the present work to examine organizational ideology is an analysis of the annual reports of two states' health and welfare agencies from 1947 to 1977.[55] The two states are Connecticut and Texas, which were also the subjects in the implementation study. Each statement of goals, whether general, organizational, or dealing with service, is noted. Trends in leadership in the agencies and external influences on the agencies are also analyzed. The annual reports provide the most consistent and permanent record of the agencies in question; because annual reports for a period of over thirty years are available, they make possible an assessment of historical trends. Such reports, uncautiously used, present pitfalls as well: they reflect only what the anonymous authors of the reports (usually the commissioners) included, not necessarily all that the agency did, or what others thought. Moreover, in addition to serving as internal records, the reports were directed to one principal external audience—the state legislatures—and this undoubtedly influenced their tone. For this reason, I supplemented and informed my detailed interpretive reading of the materials by interviews with officials of the four agencies.

In analyzing the EPSDT program in Texas and Connecticut, we shall see that it functioned effectively in Texas and relatively poorly in Connecticut. If organizational ideology were a major explanation for this difference, we should expect to find significant differences in the goals of the two states' operating agencies, and specifically that the goals of the Texas welfare agency were more nearly congruent with those of the EPSDT program than was the case in Connecticut. As it turned out, this was not the case. Ideological goals of the welfare agencies in both states proved to be similar, as were the goals of the health agencies. However, sharp differences emerged when the goals common to the health agencies were compared to those of the welfare agencies.

Welfare Department Goals

The broadest goals for welfare agencies were stated nationally by the American Public Welfare Association in 1952:

Public welfare is that area of governmental service which protects individuals and families against potential or actual social disaster, including economic want, and helps them find the means to regain economic and social self-sufficiency.[56]

With these goals as a background we can turn to Connecticut and Texas welfare agencies to assess their ideologies.

Connecticut

Connecticut stated its ideological goals in 1948 as "to conserve human resources and thus promote the general welfare,"[57] and two years later reiterated the goal as "to advance public welfare."[58]

However, broad ideological goals were not mentioned again until ten years later when a new commissioner, Bernard Shapiro, reorganized the Welfare Department and suggested that its task was "to prevent human need and to relieve it when it occurs."[59] This theme continued during the following five years, a period of expansion of welfare programs, nationally and in the state. Also added was the agency's responsibility to "join with others in assuming a leadership role in the community in seeking solutions to these many social and economic problems."[60] Thus, no longer was it sufficient for the agency to prevent and relieve human need; it was to lead others to do the same. This leadership extended not only to its clients but "to assure better living for all people in Connecticut."[61] When the Medicaid program was added to department responsibilities, the annual report noted that the federal and state enabling legislation was passed "in keeping with the existing climate of social concern and wide-spread acceptance of the opinion that access to health is a basic human right."[62]

The statements of the 1960s reflected the social climate of those years. But by the end of the decade, the state legislature and the governor's office reacted sharply against welfare spending. The progressive commissioner of the 1960s was replaced by a conservative. By 1971, agency goals were reduced: "the goal of welfare

. . . is to help people get off welfare."[63] No other goals were avowed. This tone was maintained through the 1970s, so that "one of the major goals of the Department over the last two years has been the maintenance of a caseload in which benefits are granted only to those who are eligible."[64] The operational goal of assuring that welfare assistance was limited to a narrow group of "eligibles" was a far cry from the earlier goal of helping all the people of the state. During the 1970s there were virtually no other statements of general goals. This reflected the agency's dominant concern for careful fiscal management and efficiency.

Administrative goals were discussed in nearly all *Administrative Reports* in all periods. During the 1950s the department took on increased services, set up separate units to handle finance and personnel, and established a bureau of social services to coordinate "the program and consultant personnel in public assistance, child welfare, medical and other specialties."[65] State supervision of localities was increased, with the state increasingly taking over responsibility from the localities for financing local welfare programs. During this period the agency concentrated on increasing the number of positions, hiring sufficient qualified personnel, tightening administrative procedures, and improving case handling, supervision, and staff training.[66] The department stressed uniform and efficient procedures. It wanted to extend its research and statistical capacity to compile and analyze data needed for administrative purposes; to focus on administrative needs such as adequate office space, equipment, and centralized information; and to make more efficient the method of processing payments in the child welfare program.[67] During the 1960s, as programs grew and recipients increased, the department commented on its increased responsibilities and its administrative response, particularly its Bureau of Business Administration, which was reorganized to meet growing demands.[68]

After 1971, with a predominantly conservative legislature and governor, the major administrative goals concerned efficiency:

It is the goal of your Connecticut Welfare Department to make sure that the taxpayers' money is provided only to those who are eligible for welfare, that the monies and the services provided are only those which will be of genuine benefit, and that the administration of the Department will be the most efficient and least expensive possible.[69]

These goals predominated even if it meant the contraction of the agency itself:

Until the economy improves, our goal is to manage our scarce resources as efficiently as possible. Consequently, we have started to set in motion programs which will cut costs while maintaining services to the poor.[70]

Agency personnel, which numbered 417 in 1949, reached a peak of 2171 in 1970 and then began slowly to decline to 1500 in 1976.[71] Overall expenditures continued to rise because the grant programs continued to increase in amounts. Thus, the efficiency gained consisted of a smaller staff for larger programs.

Service goals for the Connecticut Welfare Department were of two types: "to provide financial assistance to needy people,"[72] and to supervise "all children requiring the protection and discipline of the state as well as provide welfare services for children in rural areas throughout the state. . . ."[73] The bulk of the agency's time and resources was spent on financing services, not on the more direct provision of social services for children. By the mid-1950s the agency also found itself operating homes for committed children.[74] Under Shapiro's commissionership, this emphasis (at least in the reports) shifted with the recommendation that the 1956 Social Security amendments be implemented to assure "the provision of social services to public assistance beneficiaries to strengthen family life, self-support, and self-care. . . ."[75] The department, using funds from the 1962 Social Security Act amendments, was able to provide preventive and rehabilitation services for persons, including teaching people to manage their own income and to support themselves.[76] These services were characterized by the department the following year as marking "a new era of concentrated aggressive social casework approach to helping the neediest families."[77]

This era ended abruptly in 1969 when the Connecticut General Assembly voted changes in the welfare law which reduced Title XIX income levels and resources, eliminated children of unemployed parents from welfare rolls, eliminated the open-ended budget, and restricted the ability of the department to adjust assistance grants to the cost of living. The *Administrative Report* that year noted that these changes "reduced the department's ability to provide assistance through federal programs to several groups of recipients."[78]

With the change in the political environment in 1970 and the cutback in funds by the legislature, the department's involvement in the provision of social services faded from the *Administrative Reports* with the suggestion that these services might be better provided elsewhere:

One of the means by which appropriate help and services to welfare recipients might be provided more effectively and at less cost to the taxpayer is better use of resources of the private sector.[79]

The department had also begun to separate social services from financial assistance. The legislature, after much lobbying from children's interest groups, set up a separate Department of Children and Youth Services in 1974, which removed from welfare its task of caring for neglected or delinquent children.

Ironically, it was during this period of withdrawal from direct services that the Welfare Department was renamed the Department of Social Services. By 1977 social services were formally separated from income maintenance. The Department of Income Maintenance—which included the Public Assistance, Social Security, and Medicaid programs—became the larger agency, while social services were allocated to a new Department of Human Resources. Thus, the original ideological goals had by the 1970s been sacrificed for administrative goals such as efficiency, with service goals subordinate to what could be accomplished by the limited amount of funds provided by the legislature. Although during the 1960s the *Administrative Reports* were virtually advocacy reports for their clientele as much as for the welfare agency, by the 1970s they were dreary fiscal reports emphasizing decreasing fraud and abuse and increasing efficiency.

Texas

The Texas Welfare Department followed a similar pattern, but with much less variation. During the early years general social goals were related to the basic fabric of democracy:

The State Board of Public Welfare feels that the Department is making a substantial contribution to the efforts being exerted by all of Texas and America in order that our democracy shall care for its own and that it shall not perish because of a weakness from within.[80]

In child welfare, the agency saw its role as safeguarding the rights of every child who had no home, "or whose home is about to be destroyed."[81] Aside from these early comments, there were few statements of social goals in the annual reports, and they did not reappear until twenty years later. In 1972 and 1973 the format of the annual reports changed from a dry accounting of statistics to a glossy projection of an organization deeply involved in promoting public welfare and furthering broad social goals. Thus, the agency's reason for existence was "to help the people of Texas."[82] The needs of the poor of Texas were being met by state and federal programs established "to assure equitability and eligibility."[83] However, these goals were usually tempered with the limitation that the agency would meet only the "*basic* needs of certain groups of poor people."[84] This suggests an ideological two-tiered system where the Welfare Department was responsible for the welfare of only those people duly designated by the legislature. A similar limitation appeared in the Medicaid program: "In the present, DPW [Department of Public Welfare] is operating programs which are aimed to provide adequate medical care for eligible Texans."[85]

The Texas agency was constantly looking over its shoulder to see what the legislature would provide before setting out its general social goals: "We cannot forget the poor, but neither can we forget the taxpayers who pay the assistance bill."[86] With the national celebration of the Bicentennial in 1976, Welfare Department officials wrote more than usual about goals; they reflected on the growth of government involvement in welfare since the Depression, which "brought the realization that only government had sufficient command of resources and unbiased distribution mechanisms to alleviate the problems."[87]

Administrative goals appeared less frequently than they did in Connecticut reports. The one administrative item that was discussed every year was the continuing problem of keeping personnel. The Department was plagued with annual turnover rates as high as 36 percent in 1947. Only in one year did they fall below 20 percent.[88] Reports during the period also noted that Texas field-workers carried the highest case loads in the country.[89] That the high personnel turnover and the high case load might be related was never noted, although all reports commented favorably on the low administrative costs which the Texas program bore compared to other states.[90] Insofar as agencies only report what they think is important, it is clear that keeping administrative costs low was a major goal for the Texas Welfare Department whatever else might be the cost in terms of services rendered. As was noted in 1972,

"The Department's ability to fulfill the goal of social services is limited . . . by the amount of money and the number of workers available to meet demands."[91]

As in Connecticut, the Texas Welfare Department grew as more assistance programs and the Medicaid program were added and as welfare rolls expanded. Between 1949 and 1976 both personnel and expenditures of the program increased tenfold.[92]

In the 1970s the agency discussed for the first time its organization and decentralization, since greater authority was then being devolved on regional administrators.[93] The agency also established a computerized child abuse and neglect registry.[94] Two years later, regions were again redefined, and

still more changes occurred at the state office level with widespread use of the program manager concept. . . . The administration became more economical, more direct in its program delivery as a result of these and other internal innovations in 1975.[95]

The lack of discussion of administrative goals in the Texas reports does not necessarily mean that they were not important. More likely, the reports reflected a certain style of presentation. In fact, welfare officials interviewed in 1978 talked long of the concern for efficient management.[96]

Like those of Connecticut, Texas's services were of two types, financial assistance and social services. The latter, which grew out of child welfare services, frequently got short shrift because case loads were kept very high to minimize administrative costs. During the 1940s, extensive child welfare services were available to needy children in sixteen counties, but only on a limited basis in the rest of the state.[97] Over the years, these welfare services expanded to include all the rest of Texas, and by the 1950s the state was also providing welfare services to any child or any adult in any of the public assistance programs "over and above those services required to establish eligibility. . . ."[98] During the next ten years, the format of the reports remained essentially unchanged and with few new additions.

One inkling of how limited Texas's financial assistance services were during this period comes from the 1964 statement that "perhaps the most significant change during the year was the advancement of the age of children eligible for assistance under the Aid to Families with Dependent Children program from 13 years to 15 years old."[99] Presumably, children beyond the cutoff age were esteemed able to support themselves. One wonders what kind of working life awaited a thirteen-year-old with barely an elementary school education.

During the 1960s, Texas responded to federal initiatives by implementing work training and food assistance programs, and Medicaid.[100] Services increased as the welfare rolls swelled. The department saw several factors for this growth:

Among them were the normal growth rates expected because of population growth; the advent of Medicaid in Texas the previous year, providing government-purchased medical care for needy citizens and thus a new incentive to apply for public assistance under one of the Department's four categorical programs; and to some extent the U.S. Supreme Court ruling that AFDC benefits could not be denied to families with a "substitute father." Also some of the increase can be attributed to efforts of Federally funded "anti-poverty" agencies and other groups to locate potential recipients in the communities and inform them of the benefits available.[101]

As viewed by the Texas commissioner, all the factors for growth of services, except for population, were federally induced. However, the service orientation remained strong, particularly through the 1970s:

A basic function of the Department is to provide social services to children in need of protection and to their families, to AFDC recipients and to applicants and recipients of the adult assistance categories, OAA, AB, APTD.[102]

There was a major effort in children's services, including a public information program about child abuse[103] and day care licensing,[104] and even the EPSDT program received mention.[105] Even with the separation of social services from financial support programs under the federally sponsored Supplementary Security Income (SSI) program which replaced the OAA, AB, and APTD programs, the Welfare Department maintained its social services for these groups because these groups continued to "need many services they cannot afford on SSI."[106]

Thus, although the Texas Welfare Department's general social goals seemed weak and seemed to condone a purpose limited to whatever the state funds permitted and federal regulations required, by the 1970s there nevertheless appeared a concern for providing services, at least for children, even though such concern had to be expressed under a two-tier system for those in need.

Ideology of Welfare Agencies

Welfare agencies in both states seemed particularly weak in general ideological or social goals by the 1970s, if their annual reports are an accurate reflection of these goals. In terms of administrative goals, both Connecticut and Texas were concerned with efficiency. By the 1970s the service orientation of the Connecticut agency seemed weak if one read only the annual reports. However, it continued to operate more welfare services than were required by the federal government. Meanwhile, Texas's service goals seemed to be growing, too, at least for federally mandated programs.

How would these orientations affect the implementation of EPSDT, a program requiring a broad social commitment to finding needy children and providing them with care, a program requiring administrative efficiency and a strong service orientation? From the welfare agency goals one would not expect much difference in performance. If there were an ideological constraint, it should appear in both states. However, as we shall see, Texas was much more successful in carrying out the EPSDT program than was Connecticut. Thus, underlying organizational ideology does not seem to be an important explanatory factor in how these agencies performed their tasks, nor can it be argued that the orientation of the agencies served as a powerful constraint on implementation.

In both states the agencies proved to be highly responsive to policy from two sources: the federal government and the state legislature. In Connecticut, the effects of the 1956 and 1962 Social Security amendments were mentioned as the basis for implementing more social services. The effects of the federally mandated Title XX program and the splitting off of social services from financial assistance grew directly out of federal programs. The Texas Welfare Department liked to take credit for "innovations," but most often these were in fact mandated by federal law. For example, one of two innovations in 1974–1975, a state-wide transportation system, had in fact been mandated by court order because Texas had failed to provide transportation as required under Medicaid.[107]

Both states responded to the federal mandates, but they responded selectively and discussed different federal requirements, which meant they felt differently the burden of federal law. Part of the differences lay in the fact that Connecticut, throughout the period examined, had one of the more generous public assistance and Medicaid programs in the country while Texas had one of the more niggardly. This difference in itself can color responses to federal mandates. Connecticut rarely had to wait for the full force of a federal mandate to implement a particular program and often, at least until 1969, exceeded federal requirements. Texas was always operating on a minimal basis.

The concern for the approval of the state legislature appeared throughout the Texas reports. One welfare official commented about relations with the legislature in the late 1970s: "We're not very popular. Highways are more salable than welfare."[108] In Connecticut this concern appeared in the reports only after 1969, when the relationship between the agency and the legislature resembled more that of Texas, with a concern for efficiency to meet the approval of the legislature. Tensions between the agency and the legislature surfaced in 1978, when the legislature would not provide funds for what the agency considered to be adequate staff.[109]

That agencies were responsive to state legislatures is not surprising. What is more important is that in both states, welfare agencies in the 1970s were feeling strong pressures to trim their budgets and make them more efficient. Such pressures were incorporated as part of agency goals. However, despite the similarity of such constraints, the two states operated their EPSDT programs very differently, with Texas according it wide resources compared to Connecticut. Thus, the goals of the agencies *per se* did not seem to constitute an obvious constraint in implementing EPSDT.

Health Department Goals

In both Texas and Connecticut, the welfare departments were the agencies charged with responsibility to implement Medicaid and therefore EPSDT. However, due to the circumstances that there had been some debate over whether EPSDT were a health or welfare program, and that Texas chose to subcontract with its Health Department to provide EPSDT screens, a comparison might be expected to show whether or not the goals of health agencies were important in determining how the welfare agencies went about implementing the program, whether involving health agencies was a good idea, and whether having health agencies implement EPSDT would have been preferable.

In 1965, the American Public Health Association said that the purpose of public health was "to promote personal and community health, to maintain a healthful environment, and to attack disease and disability."[110] The association went on to say that it viewed state government as primarily responsible for public health within the states,[111] and that the functions of the state health agency were leadership, financial assistance to local agencies, setting and enforcing health standards, and providing certain health services.[112] The provision of personal health services was limited to areas not served by local agencies or during emergencies. Thus, health departments, despite their broader goals of promoting personal health, were not, except under unusual circumstances, to be involved in personal health services.

Both states reflected this philosophy in their annual (Connecticut) or biennial (Texas) reports. Neither state noted clear ideological goals most of the time, nor did the reports reflect a major concern with administrative growth and development. In keeping with the American Public Health Association's statements, both states concentrated on developing their capacity for regulation, supervision, and consultation, rather than direct services.

Connecticut

Connecticut in 1947 took its general social goal from the state statutes "to employ the most efficient and practical means for the prevention and suppression of disease."[113] The following year the Health Department patted itself on the back for having contributed to the substantial progress made since 1900 in protecting the health of Connecticut residents.[114] The Connecticut statutes served as the basic goals in 1949 and in later years, but the department that year also included in full a statement adopted by the American Medical Association (AMA), which defined public health as

the art and science of maintaining, protecting and improving the health of people through organized community efforts. It includes those arrangements whereby the Community provides medical services for special groups of persons, and is concerned with prevention or control of disease, with persons requiring hospitalization to protect the community, and with the medically indigent.[115]

Although broad ideological goals appeared rarely in the reports after that time, and although the AMA statement never appeared again, its basic tenets became implicit in the department's statements in later years. That the community provide medical services for special groups of persons and be concerned with the medically indigent were elements which would lead to a two-tiered system of care by which the Health Department, at least in personal health services, would be responsible for the care of only the indigent. This would assure that the department would not compete with private physicians and would distinguish clearly the roles of public and private sectors in personal health services.

In 1971, the department said in its report:

Although the primary objectives of the Department in maternal and child health are the preservation and improvement of the health of all mothers and children, *the emphasis is to provide needed services to those economically disadvantaged and socially deprived mothers and children who need them most, and receive them least.*[116]

Thus, the very broad goal of the Health Department to promote the health of the community was constrained by a narrower focus on those not cared for by the private sector. As third-party payments became available, this turned out to be a diminishing segment of the population. One other social goal of the department was health education, to motivate the public to protect itself from disease.[117]

As with general goals, one has to tease administrative goals out of the text of administrative reports because they are rarely stated explicitly. The goal of the department was to achieve full-time local health coverage throughout the state.[118] This was to be done, however, not under state control, but by encouraging localities to set up their own health departments with full-time health officers. Where there were no full-time health services, the Health Department during the 1960s set up regional offices "expanding full-time public health coverage on a regional basis, and coordinating preventive medicine programs more closely with medical care."[119]

This plan was scarcely a case of empire building because, were the venture entirely successful, the State Health Department would find its functions superseded by those of the localities. This, in fact, was the intent. Unusual as it may seem, the Connecticut State Health Department was actually attempting to diminish rather than increase its role in the delivery of health services. Aside from one reorganization in 1952 and occasional passing concern about the lack of qualified personnel in the 1960s[120] and the fact that the public health nursing division changed functions from providing direct services to serving as consultant to local agencies, there was little overall commentary on Health Department organization. The reports were filled with descriptions of many different, discrete services.

During this period, in which the nation's total health expenditures grew tenfold and the public sector's share of health expenditures grew from 25.5 to 42.3 percent,[121] the Connecticut Health Department's expenditures increased less than fourfold from $8 million in 1950 to $30 million in 1976.[122] It is difficult to interpret this growth even taking inflation into account, because the shape of the agency changed greatly during this period. In 1953, the mental health division became a separate department. In the late 1970s, mental retardation did the same, taking with it half the agency's budget. When the Department of Environmental Protection was formed, it carved out air and water pollution control. However, the Health Department received health planning functions and became the rate setting agency for hospitals and health care. Nevertheless, many of the state health functions became located outside the Health Department. The lack of discussion of administrative goals may have reflected the dearth of integral administrative or organizational goals for the department; this facilitated its dismemberment. The department's lack of involvement in public health functions was reflected in its 1967 commentary on federal legislation in health:

The last Congress passed a number of these new health laws to assure the availability and accessibility to the best health care for all Americans regardless of age, color, geography or economic status. Medicare, Medicaid, training of professionals in health and allied disciplines, additional support for research and strengthening of community health planning are examples of some of these new programs.[123]

Of the federal programs mentioned, the Health Department was responsible for administering only part of one—the community health planning legislation. Even in that legislation, the primary responsibility went to the localities. Nevertheless, the department chose to discuss these programs in its reports as if it were fulfilling a much broader function than it was in reality.

Services were the major focus of Connecticut's *Administrative Reports*, and such services came in many varieties. In the 1940s and 1950s, the Health Department's primary new goals were to establish state laboratory services[124] and to take responsibility for civil defense health services,[125] while its ongoing programs continued to be maternal and child health, crippled children, and public health nursing services.

During the 1960s public health nursing received particular attention, with a trend toward consultative rather than direct services. Whereas in 1961 the department reported that 302 expectant mothers were cared for by state public health nurses,[126] later reports noted no such direct services. By 1968, the state ended its five-year demonstration project of direct nursing services in eight towns of northeastern Connecticut.[127] Although the need for continued public health nursing was emphasized,[128] the agency function was limited to training and consultation. This shift—which took place for all personal health services—evolved from the success of the State Health Department in allocating such health tasks to local health departments and to local nursing agencies which were administratively independent of the state agency. As a later report noted:

Provision of local health services is a role the State Health Department sees itself involved in but only to the extent that it provides consultation services in the four regional offices.[129]

Thus, consultative services became the primary focus of the Health Department. Such services included surveillance for epidemics and programs in educating both the public and professionals, particularly in disease prevention:

During the year this Department initiated a number of programs aimed at reducing the gap between what is known about preventive measures in the control of chronic disease and what people do about them.[130]

It was during this period in which the health agency was shifting from direct services to consultative services that the Welfare Department began to implement EPSDT. The Health Department mentioned the program in its annual reports from 1974 to 1976, and noted its assistance to the Welfare Department in setting up the program.[131] The Health Department, however, did not provide services under the program because it could not, having phased out its service capacity several years earlier.

Regulation was also part of the Health Department's services, which included setting standards. Citing the variety of regulatory activity with which the department was involved, a report noted that in one year the department adopted or amended

regulations concerning sanitation of places dispensing food or beverages; catering food services; itinerant food vending; abortions; manufacture of ice for sale; compressed air used in self-contained underwater breathing apparatus; standards for public health nursing grants to towns having population less than 5,000, and the sale of turtles.[132]

The Connecticut Health Department seemed preoccupied with a multitude of different tasks in different areas. From its own reports, it seemed to be an agency without clear goals which deliberately kept a low profile.

Texas

In the early years surveyed (1950 to 1954), the Texas Health Department clearly stated its general ideological goals: "The prevention of disease has always been the primary purpose of the Texas State Department of Health."[133] The purpose was also to promote "positive mental health and the prevention of mental illness . . . "[134] and "to encourage, sponsor and promote dental health in Texas."[135] However, the sweeping goals "to prevent and control disease and promote positive good health" were severely limited: "At no time does the department attempt to enter the field of curative medicine."[136] By curative medicine, the department meant the private practice of medicine. This statement was an acknowledgment of the power of the Texas Medical Association, though one is hard pressed to see how a department could stay completely out of curative medicine while controlling disease.

Ideological goals became difficult to distill from the reports after the 1950s, in good part because the reports themselves rarely included an overview of the department. Rather, they listed only the activities of the various administrative divisions. Whether the ideological goals of the 1950s were carried into the 1970s cannot be deduced from the biennial reports, but health and welfare officials interviewed in 1978 indicated that the power of the Texas Medical Association continued to worry them,[137] so that broad public health goals were always tempered by a concern for the attitudes of the private sector. As we shall see in the next chapter, this led to a highly fragmented system of care.

Like Connecticut, the Texas Health Department in the 1950s was concerned with the development of local health departments.[138] By 1960 there were fifty full-time local health departments covering three-quarters of the state's population.[139] One of the problems in developing local health agencies was

the shortage of qualified local health department directors. . . . Local health departments not having the services of full-time directors have required special attention, for it has been found that public health programs can deteriorate rapidly unless directed by full-time qualified public health physicians.[140]

This statement reflected the then-prevailing philosophy that only physicians could carry out public health work. However, this philosophy was being challenged in Connecticut, which by 1970 had already appointed its first non-physician public health director. By 1968, when it became clear that many of Texas's rural areas could not be covered by full-time health department services, planning began for regionalized state health services in areas without full-time local health departments. The state was divided into ten regions and, by 1976, all of them had fully staffed operating state health services.[141] Thus, in Texas, the attempt to devolve responsibility for public health on the localities was not as successful as it had been in Connecticut, in great part because its local resources for financing and for health personnel were much more limited. The administrative philosophy remained the same: a planned abdication of responsibility, just the opposite of the expected typical bureaucratic empire-building. It is a fascinating question, but one beyond the scope of this study, to explain why these two very different health agencies adopted the same regressive behavior. Few studies have been carried out on health agencies. Most of what has been written is proscriptive rather than descriptive. The health business—and particularly the public sector—was growing so rapidly that a stance as conservative as that taken by these two states needs explanation. One possibility is that health agencies deliberately kept a low profile to avoid offending powerful organized medical interests. The fact that in Texas—and, until the 1970s, also in Connecticut—health commissioners were picked from slates presented by medical societies, would tend to confirm this view.

Nevertheless, in other areas the Texas Health Department was concerned about its own capacity to provide necessary services. In 1952 it argued strongly the need for a state laboratory, which finally was begun a few years later.[142] Department reports noted that additional funds were needed to meet mental health needs,[143] maternal and child health services,[144] crippled children's services,[145] and dental services.[146]

Efficient administration was also a concern:

During this biennium, principal administrative direction has been given to the application of sound management procedures and recognized administrative practices emphasizing clearer definitions of functions within operating divisions. . . .[147]

The department wanted to develop a sound program "in personnel administration and fiscal management."[148] Major department reorganizations took place in the late 1950s and again in the early 1970s "to reduce overlapping services and to free the time of our professional personnel by making available adequate administrative and clerical services."[149]

After the 1960s, explicit statements of administrative goals became rarer while the facts of the new organization were presented without commentary. The reorganizations reflected also the growth and increasingly complex administration of the department. From 926 in 1958–1960, the staff had grown to 4,755 in 1975–1977. Expenditures during the same period rose from $8 million to $139 million.[150] Like Connecticut, the Texas Health Department lost certain functions, such as mental health, during the 1960s (a fact not commented upon in the reports), and gained in the 1970s the state planning function under the federal Health Services Planning and Development Act. But, unlike Connecticut, it maintained functions of environmental and consumer protection. In 1975, the health agency was renamed the Department of Health Resources and for the first time health planning received first-page attention in the *Biennial Report*. However, as was typical of most of the previous reports, no overview of department activities was presented nor was there any explanation of how the new Department of Health Resources differed substantively from the earlier Department of Health. If one were to judge the department over the years from the reports, one would have to view it as a cluster of different divisions each engaged in its own discrete activity with no central link other than that all of its activities dealt with health.

Since almost all activities tended to get listed indiscriminantly in the reports, it is difficult to evaluate what were major as opposed to minor department goals. Regulation was certainly a major function in the 1950s, for what was then called sanitary engineering and food and drug administration and later called environmental health and consumer protection.

The department also carried out a large number of indirect services through consultation, for example, to local child guidance clinics,[151] or to localities on venereal disease.[152] Dental services involved "professional consultation and financial assistance to local health units, professional organizations, private practitioners, and other individuals and groups. . . ."[153] Consultation was also an important part of the Maternal and Child Health program.[154] Although the focus of these consultative services changed over time, it is hard to discern any clear trends. Throughout the period under study, a great deal of effort went into professional education programs.[155] For a period, public education was also an important goal and was a separate division in the department: "Health Education by its very nature is a major part of every program conducted by the Texas State Department of Health."[156] However, in the reorganization of the early 1970s, the public education division lost its separate status.

As part of the consultative and teaching services, the department also coordinated both public and private groups on programs, for example, on cancer and heart disease, even when they were not mandated by state statute.[157]

The Health Department provided a small amount of direct services in the Crippled Children's and Maternal and Child Health programs with diagnostic and treatment services in the former program and well-child care in the latter.[158] The Health Department added to these direct services when it contracted with the Welfare Department to provide screening care under EPSDT by establishing fifteen mobile units and subcontracting with local agencies.[159]

After 1965, the Health Department began to stress its planning functions, that its responsibilities involved "administration and evaluation of maternal and child health needs and program planning to meet these needs."[160] These planning functions increased with the establishment of a planning office and with the subsequent regionalization of the department's services. The planning role was increased when the designated State Health Planning and Development Agency mandated by federal law was placed in the Health Department in the mid-1970s.

Ideology of Health Agencies

The ideologies of health departments in Connecticut and Texas, unlike those of the welfare departments, did not develop clear trends over time. Both health agencies stated broad ideological goals only in the early days. The major goal after that seemed to be devolution of their power to local health agencies, a kind of negative empire-building. When that was not entirely successful, the state agencies provided regional services, but in Connecticut, at least, the state agency was able to withdraw after a few years. Both agencies were concerned with regulation and in later years with planning. Planning, however, must have seemed a complex procedure for the Connecticut agency when many of the public health functions were no longer in its domain. Both agencies developed a fragmented administrative structure comprising many small programs related only by some concern with health.

The ideologies of the health agencies in the two states are strikingly similar. If ideologies were predictive of behavior, one would expect that such similarities would lead to similar reactions to the opportunity to develop the EPSDT program. However, the Texas Health Department chose to contract with the Welfare Department to carry out the screening services which required a system to deliver health services throughout the state, while Connecticut's Health Department limited its participation to consultation on standards for care and on methods for attracting providers.

Is Organizational Ideology a Constraint?

From this investigation, I conclude that the organizational ideology of implementing agencies did not act as a significant constraint on the way the EPSDT program functioned in Connecticut and Texas. Although the ideologies of welfare agencies were similar in both states and those of health agencies were similar in both states, the implementation of EPSDT was, as we shall see, very different. Thus, the ideology of an agency *per se* does not seem to explain variation in program implementation. Whether a broader study encompassing more states would find evidence of differential performance that could be traced to ideology, I, of course, cannot say. With regard to the claim that ideology is an important explanatory variable predicting outcome, however, I must conclude with the judicious Scots verdict of "not proven."

One can speculate why ideology does not explain EPSDT implementation in these cases. It may be that annual reports reflect not so much what the agencies are doing, but what they hope to do. Thus, although both welfare agencies had stressed managerial efficiency and strong centralized departments, only Texas may actually have achieved that operationally. For the Connecticut Welfare Department—which had begun such management policy only in 1970—by the advent of EPSDT only a few years later, the appropriate ideology was not yet fully evident. Visits to the agencies and interviews with officials in the two states tended to support this view. The Texas Welfare Department in 1978 was an organized, efficient structure where organizational goals seemed to take precedence. The management of data systems formed an important and integral part of the administrative ethos. The Connecticut agency, on the other hand, despite great progress in its data processing systems, was always lagging behind schedules for projected improvements. There was a sense of constantly trying to play administrative catch-up.

This review of agency goals also casts some light on the issue of whether the welfare agency was a more suitable single-state agency for implementing EPSDT than health. During the period under study, welfare was growing, perhaps reluctantly, but nevertheless commanding nearly a quarter of the share of state budgets. Health saw its role as one of non-interference with the private practice of medicine and of *laissez-faire* in local affairs.

Health agencies tended toward fragmentation; their programs fled centralized direction and organizational control. By contrast, the welfare agencies were organizationally aggressive. They dealt with attacks from penny-pinching legislatures by tightening central control and searching for new and acceptable organizational missions.

During the 1970s the welfare agencies in Connecticut and Texas were simply more organizationally dynamic than the health agencies. There is no evidence that such organizational dynamism had been a factor in the federal decision in the late 1960s to assign administration of EPSDT to welfare rather than health. That decision was taken because welfare, at the federal level, had access to funds. Nevertheless, if the findings for these two states holds true for others, such a decision made good organizational sense and may have saved EPSDT from oblivion. Ideologically, welfare departments were better equipped to undertake new projects than were their counterparts in health.

5 Bureaucratic Capacity: Case Management Systems

The issue to be addressed in this chapter is whether the welfare agencies had the bureaucratic capacity to carry out the EPSDT program and, if not, whether they developed the capacity to do so. The EPSDT program presented formidable organizational tasks for the single state agencies—not tasks of extreme technological complexity such as, for example, the Polaris missile program, but nevertheless of complexity greater than usually found in a social welfare program. The management tasks including identifying children who were eligible for the program, locating them, informing them of the program, screening them (or providing for the screening), referring them for care if needed, following them up and finding them again for rescreenings as necessary, as well as arranging for transportation if requested. Most of these tasks had not been part of the Medicaid, or even the larger Public Assistance programs. For these programs, which had set welfare agencies' standard operating procedures, the agencies simply waited until their clients came to them to request services.

In order to explore this issue, I shall present first the federal attempts to provide data management assistance to the states and then examine the implementation of EPSDT in Connecticut and Texas to see how the welfare agencies met the administrative requirements for the program and whether the absence of sufficient bureaucratic capacity proved to be a constraint on program implementation. Connecticut is a state high in health resources and therefore, theoretically, should have found providers of services with relative ease, although earlier studies had shown it did not have a successful EPSDT program.[161] Texas is a large state with many children eligible for EPSDT services and with a poor distribution of providers, particularly in rural areas. However, HEW officials suggested that it had a relatively effective EPSDT case management system.[162] The in-depth case studies of each state provide insights which would have been lost in a fifty-state survey. However, one must as always warn the reader of the hazards of generalizing from a sample of two.

Federal Assistance for State Management

The management of the Medicaid program had been severely criticized by Congress in 1970: "Many States do not have effective claims administration or well-designed information storage and retrieval systems; nor do they possess the financial and technical resources to develop them."[163] To remedy this situation, Congress authorized the federal government to provide technical assistance to the states by developing a model management information system.[164] The federal government was also to provide the states with 90 percent matching funds for the cost of designing, developing, and installing mechanized claims-processing and information-retrieval systems, and 75 percent funds for the operation of such systems.[165] Since administrative costs were otherwise reimbursed at only 50 percent, Congress felt it was providing ample incentives to the states for developing such systems.

Nevertheless, states were slow to put these Medicaid Management Information Systems (MMISs) in place. This was in part due to the length of time it took HEW to develop an appropriate model system. It was also in part due to state reluctance to start any program which would generate additional costs, even if the system, when installed, was expected to save money by providing more efficient administration. Moreover, states had to expend considerable sums before they could be certified by the federal agency to receive the designated matching funds. By April 1979, twenty-five states had certified MMISs operating, and all but five states were actively planning or implementing their systems.[166]

An MMIS was designed to include subsystems to generate administrative reports as well as data on clients, services, and providers, particularly so states could monitor fraud and abuse. However, as one federal civil servant observed, the states did not always have the staffs available to analyze the monthly administrative reports which the systems generated.[167]

In 1975, when it was clear that the management model designed did not meet the needs of the EPSDT program, HEW contracted for development of a model to provide for EPSDT administration. Designing a model system, at best, is an arduous process. Three years later, this model for EPSDT information was still not completed. Meanwhile, the design had been held up by the projected revisions in EPSDT with the CHAP legislation. As the person in HEW overseeing the development of this contract said: "You can't design a system until the management of the program decides what the program is to be." [168]

The uncertainty of policy in the EPSDT program hindered the design of information systems. Hence, by the late 1970s, the states—even those with operating MMISs—lacked an appropriate way to process EPSDT data, and this was to cause serious difficulties in implementation.

As for other, less technological methods of management, such as improving staff competence through expansion and/or training, HEW provided only the usual 50 percent administrative match. However, the federal government did offer a 75 percent matching rate for EPSDT case workers. The Medical Services Administration in HEW had very limited staff of its own, and therefore could not provide much technical assistance to the states. It was only in 1975, for example, that technical assistance contracts to help states implement EPSDT were first put out to bid. Given these incentives and limited assistance by the federal government to develop state capacity, how, then, did the states do?

Connecticut

The mandate to implement EPSDT in 1972 occurred when the Connecticut Welfare Department had abandoned its freer spending programs of the 1960s and turned to an ideology based on efficiency rather than services. The Welfare Department was charged with an additional service program at a time when the legislature was encouraging it to trim costs.

Establishing the EPSDT Program

By all objective standards, the EPSDT program should not have posed great problems for Connecticut. The state had been among the top ten states in per capita Medicaid expenditures;[169] it was one of the wealthiest states in the country; it ranked high in medical resources, with 164 physicians per 100,000 population (compared to a U.S. average of 130);[170] and no area in the state was more than twenty miles from the nearest source of medical care. However, if the EPSDT program benefited from any of these factors, it was not evident in its painful and protracted implementation.

The Welfare Department sought to establish the program by working with the Health Department to help find providers of services and to develop standards of care. One must remember that at this time the Health Department was phasing itself out of providing direct services and, by 1974, had stopped co-sponsoring child health clinics in the state.[171] Nevertheless, the Health Department saw EPSDT as an opportunity for health agencies to get paid for services which had hitherto been provided free.[172] Thus, the original thirty agencies which agreed to provide services were nearly all local health nursing agencies, many of which were formerly supported in part by the State Health Department.[173] The Health Department also provided Welfare with a schedule of tests required in screening and agreed to perform lead, hematocrit, and sickle cell tests if the provider agencies themselves were not able to do so.

By the end of 1973 it was evident that local nursing agencies could not provide care to sufficient numbers of children, since only 44 percent of the eligible children lived in their districts.[174] Therefore the Welfare Department turned to private physicians, hospital outpatient departments, and neighborhood clinics. The latter two institutions were usually willing and interested in providing screening services under Medicaid, since they already served a Medicaid population. To get private physicians to participate was more difficult. Physician participation in Medicaid had never been high;[175] EPSDT screening required following certain prescribed procedures, something which did not sit well with physicians. Nevertheless, within a few years, nearly fifty physicians around the state were listed by the Welfare Department as being EPSDT providers.[176]

With a mixture of different providers, the Welfare Department was able to get sufficient coverage for children, at least in theory. The problem was how to get the children to the providers. This required a good information and data system and a system for managing cases.

Information Systems

Connecticut's Welfare Department was slow in developing its MMIS. Even as late as 1977, the department often had to hand tabulate, for example, the number of providers who participated in the program. Only in 1976 did the department hire on contract a director to plan its MMIS. Because state salaries were so low, because the private-sector reimbursement of information systems experts was so high, and because the usual civil service red tape could bottleneck appointments for months, the only way to bring someone of high caliber into the department was as a consultant, thereby circumventing civil service regulations and state salary limits.[177]

By August 1977 the department had a detailed implementation plan to submit to HEW, which finally approved it in January 1978, after some unexplained delay. The department also allocated over twenty persons to develop the program, although a long time ensued before the MMIS staff was brought up to its full complement. By early 1978 the system had been put to use for checking recipient eligibility, but projections for completion of most systems, including the administrative reports and the EPSDT component, were not even estimated, while other parts were to be completed by mid-1979.[178] As it turned out, even the basic elements of the system were not operational until 1980, while some of the subsystems were to come much later.

A new information system would not have been so necessary had not the old system been nearly useless. For many years, the state had generated annual and monthly data for inclusion in federal reports, but as one who worked with these data said: "I wouldn't want to do much more than paper a room with those FS 2082's from 1968 to 1974."[179] The Health Department had asked Welfare which handicapped children were being served through Medicaid, but was told it would have to wait at least two years before the MMIS might be able to provide such information.[180]

Thus throughout the 1970s, when EPSDT was being implemented, little help could be expected from an MMIS which was itself only in its infancy. Not being able to generate data—on who was eligible, who requested care, whether those requesting care had received it, whether those referred for care had received it, and finally to identify children in need of rescreening—left the program severely handicapped in its ability to manage cases.

Case Management

Good case management may require information (to which the Connecticut EPSDT program did not have ready access), but it also requires the resources to do the job. For the Connecticut Welfare Department, developing case management meant a continuing struggle to acquire sufficient staff and resources to manage the program. When the program began in 1973 no new staff were added. Instead, two staff persons were transferred from other tasks: one of them full time; the other, who spent 10 percent of his time on the program, was designated by the department as the EPSDT coordinator.[181]

Given these staff limitations, and given the fact that all families, when they applied for financial or Medicaid assistance, would see the intake workers at the district office, these latter workers were given the task of informing applicants of the availability of EPSDT services for children. If the parents indicated an interest they were to mail a postcard back to central offices. This constituted officially a request for services. The central office (all 1.1 persons of it) then was to send the information to the providers who were asked to find the children in question and screen them. This system had three problems: most district case workers did not know much about EPSDT and therefore could not be helpful to clients; requests stacked up in central offices and eventually were never used;[182] and most providers were not paid for doing outreach and therefore did not want to contact the child.

Because the Welfare Department had no easy way of listing children who requested care, it adopted the expedient of sending providers computer printouts of *all* the eligible children in the area. Such a system might have been acceptable to public health nursing agencies and neighborhood health centers for whom contacting children was part of their service program. Individual physicians, however, were dumbfounded when they received a stack of printouts with the names of children they were supposed to contact. One pediatrician, well known for his willingness to care for Medicaid patients, said he simply ignored the printouts. He just did not have the staff, he said, but he would be happy to care for any children the Welfare Department sent to him.[183]

As a result, Connecticut had no state-wide case management system up through mid-1977. In June of that year, the Community Health Foundation, which had contracted with HEW to give technical assistance to Connecticut as well as a number of other states, had come to the same conclusion and had noted that the state legislature "prohibits DSS [Department of Social Services] from hiring the staff necessary to run the program."[184] The department (now named Social Services rather than Welfare) well knew that staff were needed—particularly since the full-time EPSDT person had retired—and asked the legislature for funds. When these were refused, Stephen Press, Director, and Harold McIntosh, Assistant Director, of Medical Care Administration put together a proposal to use Comprehensive Employment Training Act (CETA) funds to employ twenty-nine staff to carry out outreach activities.[185] These staff joined the program in the summer and fall of 1979. In addition, the department hired a full-time EPSDT coordinator. These outreach workers could now contact families directly, help them get appointments with screening providers, and help with transportation and follow-up if necessary.

However, the staff were not permanent.[186] After a year the CETA funds would run out and the state would have to finance the positions out of its own funds. The fact that HEW would pay 75 percent matching funds for EPSDT outreach workers, as opposed to the usual 50 percent administrative match, was not a sufficient lure for the state legislature, which in 1978 again rejected the department's requests to make those staff positions permanent. The reasons for this rejection were not entirely clear to department officials, as reflected in Stephen Press's deposition in 1979; but the rejection was clearly considered to be the work of the chairman of the legislature's Appropriations Committee:

Q. Were there any studies done to see whether Connecticut could perform these services without the EPSDT workers?
Press. No, there were no studies. The chairman of . . . the Appropriations Committee was insistent that we could perform it without any staff. But, she is the only person to my knowledge that has that particular feeling.
Q. Do you know of any study that she did on the program?
Press. No, and the reality is that the federal regulations don't seem to allow us to not have staff.[187]

The Welfare Department agreed to keep the workers on until January 31, and meanwhile try to reach a permanent solution. However, by the end of November, when it was clear that the department was planning to terminate those positions, the HEW Regional Office Medicaid Director wrote a stiff letter to the Commissioner of Social Services saying: "Without these positions we feel it will be very difficult, if not impossible, for you to implement a viable EPSDT program."[188] With pressure from HEW and from a lawsuit filed on behalf of welfare clients, the state managed to find sufficient funds to make the positions permanent and even to upgrade some of them.

It had taken over six years to hire staff for the EPSDT program. Whether they were sufficient was another matter. With 29 workers for about 139,816 children who were eligible during fiscal year 1978,[189] it came out to 4,821 children per worker. Even assuming that several children were in the same family and many might not need assistance, this still seemed like a heavy case load.

Staffing was a problem not only for the EPSDT program. The entire Welfare Department was understaffed and hence demoralized.[190] Moreover, working conditions were never good: offices were crowded; supplies were low; papers and printouts often piled up on the floor because filing space was not available. As far as case management went, the department could not generate adequate information to oversee the care of the children in its charge, and it did not have adequate staff to do it manually. Not until 1980 did the program achieve the ability to ascertain which children needed a rescreening and which ones had received a physical examination through the regular Medicaid billing system. Even so, the program continued to be unable to assess what happened to children who were referred for further care.

Effects of the Management System

By having chosen to use different types of providers, the Welfare Department obligated itself to coordinate different types of care and to provide links between the system and the children and their parents. This was a much more cumbersome task than had it found a single provider to do the screening. However, because the Health Department no longer provided direct services, Welfare could expect no help from that quarter.

A second effect on the program was simply the lack of reliable information. One is hesitant to use the data presented by the department when one finds so many internal inconsistencies. The department had a particularly difficult task: to proceed with the development of a new data system while still trying to make sense of the old one. Thus it does not seem worthwhile to present in any detail the number of children screened by year in relation to the number of children eligible because until 1978 the latter was an unknown quantity, and the former included repeat screenings for the same child.

The search for efficiency in the department became all-consuming and made serious implementation of a service program extremely difficult. The bureaucratic capacity of the agency was extremely limited and the search for efficiency made for greater inefficiencies. It was not that the staff members were personally incompetent, for many were extremely hardworking and dedicated, but they were overwhelmed by the size of their task and the lack of sufficient resources.

Children did get screened—about 37,300 of them in 1978.[191] This constituted 27 percent of those eligible for care that year and 36 percent of those who should have been screened that year according to Connecticut's periodicity schedule (see table 2). However, one should keep in mind that the 37,300 figure represents screenings, not children, and since young children particularly were seen several times during a year, the actual correct number of children screened is about one-third the screenings reported.[192] The majority of children screened were being cared for, not in screening clinics, but in facilities or offices in which they could also receive the follow-up diagnosis and treatment if necessary. Connecticut in its decision to use private and public providers (physicians, hospital outpatient departments, neighborhood clinics, and public health nursing agencies), for both screening and treatment chose the open system of health services which was available to any child in Connecticut. This attempt to put Medicaid-eligible children into the mainstream of medical care failed, however, because it required management skills well beyond the capacity of the Welfare Department.

Texas

For Texas, the mandate to implement EPSDT constituted yet another federal program handed down from above. As with other federal programs before it, Texans resented the "intrusion" into their affairs. Nevertheless, they saw EPSDT as something they would have to carry out, and grudgingly they did so.

Establishing the EPSDT Program

Texas had not been among the more generous states in its welfare programs. In 1970, it spent $12.10 per capita for Medicaid compared to a U.S. average of $23.43, giving the state a ranking of fifteenth from the bottom.[193] The state had a large number of poverty areas. Out of its 254 counties, 15, with a total population of 25,000, had no physicians; 157 others, with a population of nearly 3 million, were inadequately served.[194] With these disadvantages, implementing a program such as EPSDT should have been considerably more difficult than it was in Connecticut. But this did not turn out to be the case.

Credit for getting the EPSDT program started in Texas has been given to Dr. Philip A. Gates, Deputy Commissioner for Health Policy, Planning, and Consultation in the Department of Welfare.[195] Dr. Gates decided that the only way to implement the program was to contract with the State Health Department to provide screening either through its own screening teams or through sub-contracts with the city and county health departments. In October 1972, the Welfare Department signed a contract with the Health Department, but it took until February 1973 for dental care to be-gin,[196] and March 1973 until screening began. The decision to use the Health Department was dictated in good part by the percep-tion that the local and state health departments already had the capacity to provide well-child care in areas with the most children.[197]

To carry out the program, the State Health Department set up a separate EPSDT division and developed sixteen mobile teams among the ten public health regions. Some of these teams oper-ated at fixed sites, but the others covered as many as forty coun-ties. The teams used primarily nurse practitioners, nurses, and aides. Early attempts to involve physicians as part of the teams were not successful, as the physicians could not be relied upon to attend the clinics regularly.[198] The nurses therefore were trained by, and received back-up assistance from, the regional public health physicians or those in the state offices.[199] The State Health Depart-ment also subcontracted with twelve county or city health depart-ments to provide screening. Between the mobile teams and the fixed-site clinics, theoretically, all Medicaid eligible children could be screened as needed. The major problem was transportation. Under Medicaid, the state was required to pay for transportation, and Texas, which had earlier refused to do so, by 1972 had insti-tuted a transportation program under court order. However, case workers often complained that priority for transport went to the elderly, not to children.[200]

One unfortunate result of setting up a separate EPSDT division in the Health Department was its isolation from other department activities. For example, nurses who worked in the department's regular well-child clinics could not work in the EPSDT clinics. EPSDT staff felt they were isolated and only an appendage to the Health Department.[201]

The Health Department estimated that the cost of screening per child in 1977 was $24.72 in the state-operated mobile clinics and $18.56 in the local health department clinics.[202] The department managed to minimize costs by using all its services to capacity and not allowing slack time in the clinics when there might be insufficient patients. The director of the EPSDT program estimated that a similar package of screening tests and care in the private sector would cost $92.[203]

Through this system of using only public service providers for screening, and by isolating the EPSDT program from the rest of the Health Department (the offices were, in fact, several miles apart), the Texas Health and Welfare departments built up an efficient system of delivering screening services. However, because it was a closed system, because children could be screened only in health department clinics in which they could not be treated, child health care became fragmented. Children had to be screened in one place; they had to be treated in another. Nevertheless, the program received the highest accolade from the Texas Blue Ribbon Task Force for the Evaluation of Medicaid as "the most credible component of the Medicaid program in Texas."[204] Perhaps the program's high acceptability was due in good part to its decision not to challenge the private medical sector.

Information Systems

Texas was among the first five states to have its MMIS certified by HEW in 1975. This provided the state with a means of checking eligibility and verifying claims payments. The system was quite complex, however, for although the state handled the eligibility files, actual claims processing was carried out by a contractor who acted as fiscal agent for the state. Using its computerized system, the state, for example, could identify "error-prone profiles" of persons whose eligibility might be suspect.[205] The state could also identify high utilizers of Medicaid services and inaugurate a program to avoid misuse.[206] The system was continuously being worked on and developed.

Costs for the MMIS were not easy to evaluate. The federal government by 1977 estimated it had paid Texas 90 percent of its development costs of $1.1 million.[207] Texas itself estimated its own MMIS costs for fiscal 1977 as $800,000 for development and $2.9 million for operation.[208] Whatever the exact amounts, the MMIS was a major investment which Texas was willing to make and to maintain.

The EPSDT program laid new burdens on the information system. One of the most time-consuming aspects of the development of the EPSDT program in Texas was getting approval for the data collection forms which would be used to feed to the computers. What was on the forms would determine what data there would be about the program. As a result, the Welfare Department took nearly two years to develop them. One form was to be filled out by the person carrying out the screening; a second form was to be filled out by the physician who saw a child referred for treatment; a third form was used to keep track of the case worker's contacts with a child, whether the offer of screening was accepted or refused, when contact was made, and whether screening took place and when a new contact was needed. Once these forms were in use, the Texas Welfare Department could print out monthly from its main system not only the names and addresses of those eligible, but also which children had been contacted, whether they had refused services, which ones had been screened, how many times, and which ones were due for rescreening. The data could also be generated by case workers, so supervisors in the field could see how their workers were doing.

There were some weaknesses in this system: it was only as good as the information the workers put into it, and often the workers simply knew more than the computer did. The other weakness was that the system did not tie in with the claims payment through Medicaid, so that when physicians billed for their services and did not send back a referral form, there was no way of knowing whether the treatment was due to a screening. Nevertheless, the system was far superior to that which existed, for example, in Connecticut, and it made it possible for the state to attempt a public state-wide case management system for EPSDT.

Case Management

Given a good information system, and given the state-wide network of screening clinics, the major problem in Texas was getting children to the clinics. A Texas official described the system as a sandwich: health services between two layers of social service.[209] The Welfare Department assigned to the EPSDT program from two hundred to five hundred case workers in the regional offices.[210] Each worker was given a computer printout of children eligible in his or her area and, if it were known, which ones were due for a screen. The worker was also given a certain number of appointments to fill in the screening clinics on certain dates and times. The worker then contacted the families, explained to them the benefits of EPSDT, and if they agreed to screening, made an appointment. If the family had trouble getting to the clinic, the worker arranged transportation. As often as not this meant the worker drove the family. The number of appointments made available by the Health Department determined how many children would be screened that day. Welfare officials referred to the screening appointment slots as "goals" for the case workers and felt that they provided good incentives.[211] Others suggested that such a system was impersonal,[212] and was, in fact, a "quota" system, but this was usually denied.[213] In a few areas, to supplement the welfare workers, the Welfare Department subcontracted for outreach services to community organizations, but these occasionally proved troublesome as their activities were difficult to monitor. One official worried that the agencies with superb "no-show" rates for clinic appointments might be violating the patients' rights by bringing them in against their will.[214]

The other layer of the welfare sandwich was for the case workers to follow up their clients and assist them in making appointments with physicians if they were referred from the clinic. This proved more troublesome for the workers. Referrals officially were to be made from central offices (where a physician would verify the need for referral). Central offices would then inform the case worker who would then contact the clients. However, screening teams would sometimes let the referral forms stack up.[215] Case workers were often frustrated by the slowness of the referral system and, not infrequently, both the screening clinic and the case worker would essentially agree on a referral even without the decision having been formally taken by a physician in central offices.

Case workers also had trouble finding physicians for clients. Physicians were hostile to Medicaid. They testified that they were not participating in the program because of red tape and low payments.[216] Even when physicians agreed to see the Medicaid-eligible children referred from clinics, they often refused to fill out the special referral forms. This meant that the case worker had to verify treatment by contacting either the provider or the client, and then submit his or her own form. One physician, who had seen a child referred for a heart murmur, anemia, and ear infections, was so incensed by the forms that he provided no information on how or whether the child had been treated, but covered the form with his criticisms of the Medicaid program.[217] Despite these difficulties, when the Welfare Department surveyed children referred during three months of 1977, it found that an encouraging 82 percent of the children referred had been treated.[218] Whether this is a sufficient rate, when one considers that screening without follow-up is worthless, is a good question, but at least Texas, unlike Connecticut, could identify what types of services it was providing to whom.

One additional problem for the system was the outreach form on which the case worker noted when clients were contacted, whether services were requested, and when screenings and referrals took place. The data generated by this form were only as good as what the case workers fed into it. Thus, case workers and their supervisors found that the printouts usually ended up telling them only what they already knew. It was almost as if the system were being developed just to generate data, not to facilitate better services to children.

Costs for the outreach workers and administration ran high. The best estimate was that it cost about $40 per screen.[219] Such high costs would not endear the program to the legislature, and although it survived unscathed the Blue Ribbon Task Force Review in 1977, it did not survive intact the FY 1978 budget of the legislature.

In FY 1978, the legislature cut the EPSDT program by 10 percent. Compared to cuts elsewhere in the Welfare Department, the program did not fare badly, but such cuts were sure to affect the program. Two major changes resulted. In central welfare administration, the team which had developed the EPSDT case management system was broken up and each person assigned to different tasks under a functional rather than programmatic organization. The second effect was the loss of case workers for EPSDT. The exact number lost was not available, because it was said that the workers would be given generic rather than programmatic assignments. One supervisor noted, however, that her case workers had declined from eighteen to six, and that those who remained would have no time to follow up their clients.[220] Simultaneously, the Health and Welfare departments lowered the targeted number of children they expected to screen annually, although they also benefited from the fact that the number of children who were eligible had declined moderately. Thus the elaborate organization for case monitoring that had been built up over the years was being routinized. Whether this would eventually affect the quantity of EPSDT services could not, of course, be assessed for several years.

Effects of the Management System

There were two effects of Texas's case management system. The first was that a large number of children received screening services through EPSDT. In 1978, one-third of all those eligible received screening services as did 60 percent of those who should have been screened that year, according to the state's periodicity schedule (table 2, p. 49). This is an impressive achievement considering the dearth of health resources in the state and considering the transportation problems.

The second effect of Texas's case management system was to create a highly fragmented system of health care services for Medicaid-eligible children. Children could not be referred for immunizations because this was not a referrable condition under Texas Medicaid regulations. The Health Department operated separate immunization clinics and well-child clinics, but these were kept apart from EPSDT clinics and the personnel did not mix. The three clinics might be held at the same site but on different days or at different hours. Since EPSDT allowed only an annual screen, some EPSDT clinic nurses recommended to mothers of infants that they take their children to well-child clinics so they could be seen more often during their first year, as the Academy of Pediatrics recommended. However, others discouraged this pattern. EPSDT clinics were not allowed to treat for any conditions, even minor ones such as prescribing Kwell for scabies, even though about three-quarters of what was seen in the clinics could be treated by the nurses.[221]

The explanation for this fragmentation given was the concern for the Texas Medical Association. As one official put it, "a diagnostic and treatment program would have been unacceptable to the Texas Medical Association."[222] The fragmented system had been established to avoid threatening private physicians, not necessarily to meet the needs of poor children. Thus Texas had created a very successful case management system and succeeded in screening a large proportion of its eligible population despite great odds; but the costs had been high, both financially and in terms of the quality of care rendered.

Is Bureaucratic Capacity a Constraint?

The answer to this question is "yes" for Connecticut and "no" for Texas. Connecticut had been unwilling to invest in an information system, and the one that it finally started building was not ready in time for the EPSDT program. Moreover, the legislature was unwilling to finance the case workers necessary to carry out the program. Without the staff and without the information system, and with the decision to operate within the open system of multiple public and private providers of health services, the program could barely function. Moreover, it proved impossible to evaluate just how it was functioning. Texas, with its excellent information system, and with the willingness to finance case workers (at least until 1978), was able to develop a state-wide network of screening services.

The bureaucratic constraint was overcome relatively easily in Texas by the simple expedient of money. Although Connecticut was spending more per capita on Medicaid than Texas, it would not spend it on the EPSDT program or on the administrative costs needed to build capacity. There does not seem to be anything intrinsic to welfare agencies which prohibits them from carrying out programs of this sort given the necessary resources. The Texas State Welfare Department demonstrated that, given a chance, it could put together a very credible program.

One conclusion from these two experiences is that states such as Connecticut with relatively generous welfare or social programs do not necessarily build the bureaucratic capacity to manage them well. Texas had emphasized its capacity and built its competence in managing a program of the complexity of EPSDT while providing only limited benefits to its clients. Certainly it is possible for states to manage well and also provide ample services, but these are expensive policies. The EPSDT experience in Texas indicated that despite the program's complexity, it was not beyond the capacity of a state willing to invest in it. The question, then, is: Why did Texas invest and not Connecticut? One possible reason is that in Texas, with its poor network of health resources in rural areas, EPSDT was viewed as less of a threat and therefore could garner more support from the state legislature. In Connecticut, implementation of any public system threatened established private systems. Nevertheless, Texas's system of administration was acceptable only so long as the delivery system remained fragmented and did not challenge private physicians.

Institutional Constraints

From the examination of three institutional constraints in this and the preceding two chapters, it becomes evident that none of them necessarily hinders program implementation. Federal-state relations proved the most troublesome for the EPSDT program because of the inability of federal policy to prevail in the states. Whether one takes a cooperative or coercive model of federal-state relations, it is difficult to explain state and federal behavior. States did not behave in the cooperative manner which the matching-fund relationship would suggest. They resisted as much as they could what they saw as impositions from on high. If anything, states saw the existence of the program as coercion. However, when one examines HEW's inability to enforce the penalty, the coercion model does not seem appropriate, either. More likely, there were different and conflicting sets of values at federal and state levels; probably, each of the forty-nine states with a Medicaid program also had its own set of values.

However, as we have seen, the federal values for EPSDT were themselves ambiguous and beclouded. This made it easier for state values to prevail or, at least, to lessen the impact of the federal program. Lack of clarity is typical of much federal policy and that, rather than the character of the federal-state relationship in itself, may prove to have been the insuperable constraint.

Although implementation of EPSDT differed notably in Connecticut and Texas, the ideologies of the welfare agencies in the two states differ little one from the other; likewise, the health agencies resemble one another. We can identify one ideological culture for the welfare agencies, and another for the health agencies. Significantly, the welfare agencies—at least in these two states—are bureaucratically dynamic, while health agencies are not. If this finding can be generalized, it would be an important consideration when planning responsibility for health programs.

Bureaucratic capacity seems to be entirely dependent on a state's willingness to invest sufficient funds. It is not an insuperable constraint, merely one that depends on the value states set on developing it. Moreover, since building capacity takes time as well as money, it is scarcely a constraint that can be overcome overnight.

Conservatives would argue that the responsibility for social programs should be given back to the states. Such an argument assumes that what Congress did was irrelevant and that only state values should prevail. The problem with this thinking is that it excludes the possibility for national values to prevail over state values. Moreover, it assumes that states, if left to their own devices, would solve social problems such as health care for poor children. When one reviews the history of social programs in the United States there is little to support such a sanguine view of the states' social conscience. Almost every federal policy was developed in response either to the lack of such policy within the states or to the inequities among state policies. In the case of health programs, to abandon such programs to the states would be to abandon the national value of equitable health services for children. Congress may choose to do so, but many state governments, confronted by a loss of federally financed social programs, will probably object even more strongly if they are left to shoulder alone the cost and responsibility of social progress than they do when they can share the burden with the federal government. Under such conditions, equitable health and social welfare programs would be unlikely to survive.

III The Technological Constraint: Is There a Consensus?

Since medicine is the compendium of successive and contradictory errors made by doctors, when one summons the best of them, one has a great chance of requesting a truth which will be acknowledged as false a few years later. Thus, to believe in medicine would be the supreme folly if not to believe were not an even greater one.

Marcel Proust, *The Guermantes Way*

Who shall decide, when doctors disagree?

Alexander Pope, *Moral Essays*

Searching for a Consensus on Standards for Child Health Care

Doctors do often disagree. Indeed, such disagreement is an essential engine of scientific progress. However, fundamental disagreement about goals and strategies can be accomodated only with great difficulty within large-scale bureaucratic programs. EPSDT was a complex bureaucratic program which already had its share of enemies for reasons having nothing to do with its scientific rationale. It would have additional difficulty if there were not consensus in the scientific community about the merits of preventive health care and screening, the medical techniques on which the program was based.

Defining Terms

EPSDT was potentially a comprehensive health care program for poor children. The drafters of the law had used the terms "early and periodic screening, diagnosis, and treatment." Periodic screening was understood to include the preventive, health maintenance, or health supervision component of the care rendered. It was modeled after the case finding of Crippled Children's Program. The inclusion of all three functions of medical care, (screening, diagnosis, and treatment) meant that comprehensive care was an integral part of the intent of the legislation. This is the way the term "comprehensive care" has been used in this study. Others have provided more elaborate definitions including family, psycho-social, nutritional, and even recreational care.[1] Comprehensive care is easily confused with primary care which also involves preventive, diagnostic, and treatment care, usually at a single site.[2]

Primary care is usually focused on the physician or his substitute who has responsibility for providing and following up care.[3] In fact, the more one examines primary care, the more difficult it is to distinguish it from comprehensive care: "Primary care must be comprehensive . . . provide continuity of care . . . provide for coordination . . . must be patient and family centered . . . a multiprofession interdisciplinary function."[4] Comprehensive care has one element lacking in primary care. Because the former encompasses social services, it may include care-giving institutions which reach out to clients in the community.

Both comprehensive and primary care encompass prevention, screening, health maintenance, and health supervision. Some or a great deal of prevention, such as sanitation, nutrition, or the act of not smoking, may be outside the scope of comprehensive care. What remains in personal health services is known as preventive medicine. Preventive medicine is what physicians do to preserve health. It is a limited field compared to the scope of other medical services, and generally has been relegated by the physicians to low status.[5]

Health maintenance and health supervision, terms which may be used interchangeably, are the activities carried out by physicians and their associates to preserve health. Health maintenance as a word has had a particular vogue since it was adopted as the code word for prepaid group health organizations. It should be added that individuals themselves, without benefit of physicians, may also carry out health maintenance.

Screening, the technology specifically mentioned in the 1967 Child Health Act, means either a single test or a series of tests which can be administered quickly, harmlessly, and inexpensively with a high degreee of validity and reliability to ascertain whether a person has a disease or condition for which care is known and available. Definitions have varied somewhat over the years, with some confusion arising from whether cost-effectiveness should be a criterion and what degree of reliability and validity is required for the tests. Three sets of criteria are involved: those having to do with the test, with the disease, and with social, personal, and economic costs.[6] Very few, if any, types of mass screening programs meet all the necessary criteria. W. W. Holland, for example, concluded after the *Lancet*'s survey on screening that mass screening was hard to justify for any condition save phenylketonuria (PKU).[7] Nevertheless, screening remains a popular form of preventive health care and may be useful for selected groups of people. EPSDT screening, for example, is a series of tests and is therefore more of a mass periodic health examination than a mass screening program.

If we accept these definitions, we can say that the EPSDT program was a program designed to provide comprehensive care for Medicaid-eligible children. It required providers to reach out and bring children in for care, to provide health supervision, and provide primary care through screening, diagnosis, and treatment. That the EPSDT program never operated in such a comprehensive fashion was due as much to the confusion among health professionals as to how all the pieces fit together, as it was due to either the incrementalist vision of its framers or institutional constraints.

Origins of the Periodic Health Examination

The history of health care can be viewed as a struggle between the proponents of health preservation and the proponents of the healing arts. For much of this history, healing has seemed the dominant force. Hygeia, the goddess of health, became a member of lesser importance in the household of Aesculapius, the great healing doctor in the pantheon of the Greeks and the Romans.[8] Since then the medical profession has tended to relegate preventive medicine to a small corner of its field while leaving the vast area of public health to be handled by other persons. The major innovations in health preservation, such as sanitation in the nineteenth century, were made long before the germ theory was properly understood. Moreover, they were carried out by public or voluntary services, not necessarily by the medical personnel of the day. However, during the late nineteenth century curing became increasingly acceptable as the dominant segment of health preservation and care. Prevention of disease became primarily the domain of the public sector, with local health departments, national agencies, and voluntary organizations taking on the job of detecting infectious disease, searching for its cause, and organizing society for the attack on these diseases. This dichotomy between Hygeia and Aesculapius, between preventing and curing, became blurred by the beginning of the twentieth century with the addition of a third force in health: screening for non-symptomatic diseases. This early detection process arose as a result of technological innovation and progress.[9]

These technologies increased the activities of the medical profession, increased the costs of medical care, and raised intimations of immortality in the public mind.[10] Early technologies included x-rays for screening for tuberculosis, stethoscopes for detection of heart murmurs, and the Papanicolaou test for the detection of cervical cancer. Today, the list of conditions which can be screened for is long.

Originally, most screening programs were established mainly to protect the public from persons who unknowingly had infectious diseases.[11] These procedures more often benefited the screener than the screened, since little treatment was available for the infectious persons, who then found themselves segregated as well as sick.[12]

The periodic health examination developed simultaneously with the technologies for screening. Such an examination involved a combination of screening procedures as well as the compilation of a health history. The periodic exam was generic, not disease or condition specific. Although it had been suggested as early as 1856, the annual exam found its first true support in the 1920s through the confluence of interests of insurance companies and the medical profession.[13]

In 1922 the American Medical Association voted to promote periodic examinations and issued a handbook delineating what should be included in the exam. With the National Health Council, it informed the public of the need for periodic or even annual physical examinations.[14] If the campaign failed, it was partially because there were not enough physicians available and partially because the periodic medical examination did not fit into the training and practice of most physicians at the time.[15]

However, the periodic examination did receive official sanction of a sort when preventive medicine was incorporated as part of the recommendations of the Committee on the Cost of Medical Care in its report in 1932.[16] The goal remained for every person in the United States to have a periodic physical examination. Oddly enough, it took thirty years for that well-established tradition to be evaluated for effectiveness. The results were, at best, mixed, and became increasingly discouraging as time went on.

Industrial studies conducted in the 1950s showed that periodic examinations benefited the employees because they detected previously unsuspected conditions in about one-third of those examined.[17] Later studies noted the proportion of previously undiscovered diseases rising as high as 55 percent of those examined.[18] The industries involved were for the most part enthusiastic about the results.[19] However, only a few of these studies assessed the actual results from periodic examinations in terms of prolonged longevity or lessened mortality.[20] No doubt, more diseases were being found in examinations, but it was not clear whether finding these diseases led to treatment and cure, or whether persons just learned to live with something they had previously been able to ignore and about which, in any case, they could or would do nothing.

The major study which supported the periodic examination was undertaken by the Kaiser-Permanente Group Health Plan in northern California. In a nine-year follow-up of study subjects who were encouraged to have multiphasic periodic examinations,[21] and control subjects who were not, the former group had a significantly lower mortality than the latter group for one "preventable" disease, colo-rectal cancer.[22] These findings, relating to only one disease, however, were then taken to justify the continued use of periodic health examinations.

The periodic exam as a form of multiple screening has aroused passionate debate. As Sackett and Holland pointed out, the screening advocates and the methodologists were arguing not different sides of the same question but entirely different questions. One side was asking whether screening were good or bad, while the other side was asking whether there were any scientific basis for making screening decisions.[23] Results indicating that the diseases which eventually caused death were identified in only 51 percent of persons having had a health exam during the previous year spurred on researchers not to question the value of the periodic health examination, but to improve the diagnostic procedure.[24]

However, a five-year follow-up of insurance company employees suggested that even the psychological reassurance that people receive following such checkups was ill-founded, since researchers uncovered several cases of persons dying from undetected illness shortly after the examination.[25] By the mid-1970s the skeptics were beginning to outnumber the believers, and even the believers had modified their original stance to suggest less frequent than annual examinations.[26] The public also received its first taste of contradictory opinion when a physician published a strongly reasoned argument against physical examinations in the Sunday *New York Times Magazine*.[27] Although some said that the periodic examination would have to be continued merely because the public wanted it as a right,[28] this "right" had, of course, been established as a need by the very medical professionals who were now beginning to disown it.

The story of the periodic health exam had in fact begun to come full circle: physicians who had earlier been the most significant backers of periodic health assessments had begun to move away from them. Where they did support them, it was found that, for the most part, such examinations could be carried out by non-medical personnel such as physician associates and nurse-practitioners. The flush of interest in periodic exams had been fostered by the strong beliefs in the efficacy of a technology and the converging interests of the medical profession and insurance companies. The period of disillusionment set in with the recognition that the technology was not necessarily capable of detecting disease sufficiently early to alter its natural course.

Thus, one major weapon in the medical arsenal of prevention, the periodic health examination, was no longer considered as potent as it once was. Nevertheless, the exam persisted and no doubt will continue to be used, even though its original supporters lost enthusiasm. The exam continued because prevention and periodic medical care are attractive, low in cost, and appear harmless. These beliefs may operate quite independently of whatever concrete values periodic or preventive care may have. The strong interests and beliefs associated with preventive medical care were independent of any medical value it had. These beliefs included the right to medical care and the equal rights of access regardless of income. Such beliefs account for the persistence of policies even when their original supporters begin to disown them.

The periodic medical examination was attractive also because it provided a link between the warring forces of health, Hygeia and Aesculapius. Hygeia's needs for prevention were met through the ministrations of Aesculapius, the healer. The alliance was an uneasy one.

Special Risks and Needs of Children

The movement toward preventive child health services must be viewed within the context of this larger national trend. The proponents of preventive services had a number of arguments favoring special care for children, the main ones being that (1) children were a particularly high-risk group with special needs, (2) children were a valuable investment as future workers and soldiers, and (3) preventive services seemed especially effective for children.[29]

That children were a group with special needs was perceived by the late 19th century. Public officials and physicians concentrated on improving the infant's lot and instructing mothers in appropriate hygiene, and in the use of pure water and milk.[30] It was sufficient to look at infant and child mortality rates to conclude that infants and children were bearing an unequal burden of ill health in the population. Some infants were worse off than others: as early as 1918, black infants had been shown to have morbidity and mortality rates nearly twice those of white infants.[31]

Infectious diseases gave the infant mortality rate seasonal peaks, during the winter from pneumonia and during the summer from intestinal diseases. By the early 1920s the risks of poor nutrition were also known and publicized. The action of Vitamin D in preventing rickets made it clear that certain illnesses affected only children and were of grave consequence to their future.[32]

The idea that children had health needs different from other segments of the population received official recognition in 1922, when Congress passed the Sheppard-Towner Act, which provided the first federally funded public health or welfare services to be made available to the states.

The hazards of the birth process and infectious diseases eventually began to come under control; yet children continued to be viewed as a special high-risk group, although the focus of the illnesses changed. Thus by 1935 handicapping conditions called for special attention for children including, of course, rehabilitation from polio, whose incidence had continued to rise while those of other infectious diseases were declining.[33]

Although rheumatic fever and leukemia were viewed as increasing hazards for children, the infant mortality rate still offered the most dramatic evidence of need among children. In 1949, the American Academy of Pediatrics noted that "From Pearl Harbor to V-J Day 281,000 Americans were killed in action. During the same period 430,000 babies died in the United States before they were a year old—3 babies for every 2 soldiers."[34]

Infant mortality rates became the favorite rallying cry for children's needs. Although the rate had declined from 69 deaths per 1,000 live births in 1925–1929 to 25 per 1,000 in 1964, it was still considered too high; in the same period, Sweden had succeeded in lowering its rate to 14 per 1,000.[35] Chronic handicapping conditions were also noted as needing attention.[36] Most important, however, was that certain children, those living in poverty, were singled out for special attention. Increasingly, people drew attention to the lower mortality of white middle-class children compared to those children who were poor or black, or both. Although both black and white children had benefited from declines in mortality rates, the disparity between black and white rates remained.[37]

Thus the earlier concerns for the risks of all children were gradually replaced by concern for the risks of certain children. These high-risk poor and minority children were identified as those with high mortality rates, a high proportion of untreated chronic illness, and low access to preventive and medical care.[38]

The second reason for giving priority to children over other population groups was that children were viewed as the future workers of the country. Hence, their health was viewed as an asset for the common good. As a pediatric journal noted in 1908: "The future value of the child depends upon his health. . . . Will the state allow these conditions tending towards a degenerate race or will it insist that the child shall be raised properly, and become a support, not a burden?"[39] The experience of the high number of rejectees for the draft during World War II and during the 1960s indicated that poor health was depriving the country of manpower.[40]

The third reason for targeting preventive health services on children was that these services seemed to be especially effective for them. This belief appears to have been sufficient of itself, without the proof of its effectiveness being necessary.[41] As noted earlier, the consequences of preventive action were not always clearly agreed upon or understood. The debate surrounding periodic health examinations had had its repercussions in child health. Nevertheless, two types of interventions for children had generally been greeted with great enthusiasm and acceptance by the medical and other health professions, and more slowly but steadily by the lay public as well.

The first of these were the interventions against infectious and nutritional diseases. Since these techniques arrested a disease before it appeared, they constituted what was known as primary prevention and formed what were believed to be the most effective group of measures. Generally, they cost less than other types of care, and involved either removing the source of infection or disease from the individual or developing an individual's resistance to it. For example, rickets, from which perhaps nearly half the poor urban child population suffered, could be controlled with heavy doses of sun and cod liver oil.[42] The cost of both was minimal. More expensive were interventions to protect children from pellagra, which was found to be directly tied to family income. Nevertheless, during the Depression, the Farm Security Agency assisted farmers in home food production, recognizing that adequate nutrition affected resistance to this and other diseases.[43]

The protection afforded against illness by the development of sanitation, better housing, and better nutrition was encouraged by the introduction of classes for mothers.[44] Finally, and perhaps most important in dealing with infectious diseases, was the development of immunizations. Although smallpox vaccination had been known since the eighteenth century, by 1930 only 21 percent of urban children and 7 percent of rural children had been vaccinated.[45] Nevertheless, with the development of diphtheria antitoxin, the mortality rate from that disease declined from three hundred per thousand in 1900 to less than one hundred per thousand by 1920.[46] Similar experiences followed with tetanus, pertussis, polio, measles, and rubella immunization campaigns, which convinced health officials that immunization was one of the most effective ways of preserving the health of children.

The second type of generally acclaimed intervention for children was secondary prevention, screening for particular conditions or diseases. The assumptions underlying this practice were, first, that diseases or conditions discovered early in their course would be curable, or at least more responsive to treatment than those discovered when they were already symptomatic; and second, that children in particular suffered serious developmental setbacks when diseases or conditions were not promptly discovered and treated. In the first case were diseases such as rheumatic fever, which could be avoided by prompt treatment of streptococcal infections with antibiotics.[47] In the second case were vision and hearing impairments, which when untreated could lead to retarded learning by children who could not hear or see properly to comprehend what was being taught.

Screening for genetic diseases, which became feasible by the 1960s, permitted discovery of diseases early enough to prevent handicapping. Prenatal screening for Tay-Sachs, an incurable and inevitably fatal disease found predominantly among descendants of Eastern European Jews, could permit parents to decide whether or not they wanted to carry infants to term. If parents were screened before they conceived, they could decide whether they wanted to have children at all.[48] Phenylketonuria (PKU) was a particularly successful case of screening. Detection of the genetically-linked metabolic deficiency shortly after birth led promptly to the appropriate diet that prevented retardation.[49]

The merging of these screening tests resulted in a package of

tests known as the well-child exam, the well-child conference, preventive health checkups, or the child health exam. For children,
the periodic health exam grew not only out of the adult periodic
exam, but also out of the pure milk movement, which after 1912
began to measure and examine the babies as well as to promote
breast-feeding and to educate the mothers when they visited the
health station.[50]

The child health examination combined measurements of height
and weight, health histories, developmental assessment, vision
and hearing screening, and a certain number of laboratory tests for
anemia and bacteriuria, depending on the particular era and the
person doing the exam. In contrast to attitudes toward adult exams, not only was the belief in preventive visits for children a
firmly held dogma, but that segment of the public which could
afford medical care accepted it as practice. Periodic checkups were
viewed as "the backbone of pediatric practice."[51] By 1949, 54 percent of pediatric visits were for well-child care.[52] Twenty years later
the proportion had not substantially changed according to one
study,[53] although another study reported that only 36 percent of
visits to pediatricians were for well-child care. For general practitioners and internists, however, the proportion of preventive visits
was lower, 25 and 14 percent respectively.[54] Although the ideal
model may have been for well children to be seen regularly in physicians' offices, this policy tended to be carried out only in pediatricians' offices which were clustered in suburban and well-to-do
urban areas.

Only in the 1950s did this article of faith—that well-child visits
lead to better health—begin to be tested, and then only tentatively.
The results were not encouraging to believers in preventive care,
but not sufficient to dampen their ardor. The major question addressed was whether process affected outcome. Did the fact of
having well-child visits actually improve the health of children? In
a study following school children from the first through fourth
grades, the routine annual school exams were found to be of little
value for finding previously unknown diseases or conditions.[55]
Similar findings were reported for the routine physical examination of infants under a year old.[56] Whether infants had three or six
preventive visits during their first year seemed to make little difference, as did whether they were seen routinely by pediatricians
or nurse practitioners.[57] Most of these studies concentrated mainly

on yield or utilization outcomes, as opposed to whether preventive care prevented morbidity and mortality. This is difficult to measure, for children as well as adults. However, even when morbidity was measured, no differences could be found between those children receiving preventive, continuous, comprehensive care and those not receiving such care.[58]

Whether the special effectiveness of prevention for children can be documented is debatable. Some types of prevention, such as those dealing with nutrition and infectious diseases, were well accepted as effective in public opinion and medical literature. Other types of intervention, involving early presymptomatic identification of diseases, had also had a large following both professionally and among the lay public, and their effectiveness had been questioned only occasionally.

Prevention remained a major concern. Children, however, not only were no longer the focus, but were frequently ignored. When the New York Academy of Medicine in 1974 held a symposium on *Prevention and Health Maintenance Revisited*, children, their needs, and prevention's particular effectiveness for them were not mentioned in any of the papers.[59]

Although prevention may have received renewed attention, the effectiveness of preventive measures, at least for children, was becoming less and less clear. Many of the major preventive measures had already been taken to preserve child health. Whether further steps such as periodic visits, genetic screening, and others could yield more than marginal returns was beginning to be a matter of concern to those who had been setting standards and criteria for care.

Search for Consensus on Standards

For preventive care, as for treatment, the medical profession seeks to ascertain the validity and efficacy of its actions. This, at least, is its goal, and for a long time it was believed that the criteria for most preventive measures fell within its domain.

In preventive health care, the purpose of setting standards is twofold: first, to ascertain the minimum care necessary to preserve, maintain, and restore health; and second, to control the costs of health care. There have been sufficient pronouncements on the need for preventive health care—the need for well-child visits, the need for immunizations—that it is not an unreasonable exercise to look for standards for these activities. Setting standards presupposes that the factors contributing to health are known. Knowledge, however, is not perfect.

Although much has been written about the quality of health care, less attention has been directed to the minimum standards needed to maintain health. This creates problems. Writers on quality assessment start off with the question: Given certain diseases, disease processes, symptoms, or conditions, what are the best ways of diagnosing and treating them? This approach is limited by the choices already made as to what diseases or conditions are worth examining. Often, those chosen are not necessarily those which have the greatest impact on health, but those which seem most amenable to measurement. In general, the methods have been of high quality and the reviews of results careful and thoughtful.[60] However, the problem with the technique is that it fails to ask the more difficult question: What are the procedures necessary to safeguard health and are these all within the medical domain?

The second problem with the quality assessment approach is that it is based upon the assumption that there are in fact clear disease identities. Either one has a disease or one does not. However, particularly in chronic diseases, the most frequent case is that in which one has a little bit of it. How much of it is enough to be harmful? How much of it is necessary for treatment to be indicated?[61] The cutoffs chosen for defining disease, though not entirely arbitrary, are not perfect. Thus, it is generally recognized that the proportion of poor children with iron deficiency anemia in Baltimore might have been lower than the one-third reported in Kessner's study, had the criteria for anemia been set at a hematocrit lower than the 34 or 35 percent (depending on age) established by the evaluators.[62] Since some physicians may not treat children until their hematocrits fall below 33 percent, this latter criterion would not have been unreasonable.

With these drawbacks, it is not surprising that much public and private energy has been invested in the process of developing criteria solely for treatment of disease rather than the preservation of health. The former are easier to evaluate and to develop. Certainly, in pediatrics, the development of criteria for the preservation of health has been an uncertain and not always happy project.

Who is Responsible for Children?

The search for consensus on standards for child health care is bound up with a search for understanding who is responsible for child health. When public decisions are made in an open system, and when government finances health care, then the issue of responsibility becomes important. Those who determine the type of care and determine who shall deliver it are likely to be the ones to benefit from a government program.

Responsibility for child health care can be discussed on the philosophical and on the institutional levels. The philosophical debate on the responsibility for child health has centered on the tensions between the family and the state. The assumption has been in the United States that, ultimately, the family is responsible for a child's health, but if at any time the family were unable to shoulder the responsibility, the government could step in. As the head of the Children's Bureau, Grace Abbott, once noted: "All children are dependent, but only a relatively small number are dependent on the state."[63]

The federal government has been ambivalent about its responsibility for child care: "non-intervention in the generality of parent-child relationships was formally affirmed as a public value early in the century and affirmed again in the recent past."[64] Federal legislation for child health has always been careful to direct itself only to those children in special need. With the increase of federal funds and programs for child care (Head Start, AFDC, Child Welfare), and with changes in the social environment during the 1960s, social critics voiced concern that responsibility for the child had been taken from those closest to the child, the parents. The parent became a "coordinator, without voice or authority. . . ."[65]

To counteract this trend, two reports issued in 1976 and 1977 identified the family as the institution that needed support to promote the health and welfare of children.[66] Ironically, both reports called for more government intervention, although its purpose was to support the family unit as a whole rather than the child as an individual.

The focus of dependency had changed since Grace Abbot noted that all children were dependent. By the mid-1970s, not only were children perceived as dependent, but some families as well. This dependency was seen, however, not as a result of a change in philosophy, but because of private-sector market failures. The government was only to step in where other resources were lacking. As C. Arden Miller noted,

But insofar as these [private] incentives fail, government must assume a responsibility to provide medical care—from local government if possible and from federal government as necessary. In matters of children's health government must become the residual guarantor for services.[67]

Thus, philosophically, the family remained ultimately responsible for a child's health and welfare in America. Only if that system failed was society, in the form of governmental institutions, allowed to protect the child.

The second level on which the debate over responsibility for child health took place was on the practical level of institutional control. If public decisions were to be made about child health, who should make them? Should they be made by pediatricians as individuals or in groups, by other physicians, by child health advocates, government bureaucrats, education specialists, or by whom? In health care, who was responsible for the child? Who should set standards for child health care?

At this level of debate, public decisions may be made not only for those children for whom the state is the residual guarantor of care, but for other children as well. For example, standards for day care programs may be necessary for publicly sponsored programs, but these standards may become regulations that are then applied to both public and private day care centers. Thus, although the need to make decisions is triggered by those children for whom the state is responsible, these decisions affect other children as well. Hence the widened importance of such debates.

Pediatricians have been in the center of this debate on child health standards. For the most part, they have viewed themselves as responsible for standards, but without sufficient authority to fend off incursions by less qualified persons or groups. Their responsibility has been stated not in absolute terms, but in relation to other groups or individuals. Three groups have challenged pediatricians in their assertion of responsibility: the government, educators, and other physicians.

Early on, the American Academy of Pediatrics viewed the federal Children's Bureau as having overstepped its original narrow investigatory role. The pediatrician considered himself the only one qualified to lead, as the president of the academy noted in his address of 1936: "However, the laity are dominant in the control of these [child welfare] movements, and it is high time for the pediatrician to take his proper place at the head of the procession."[68]

A major source of irritation to the Academy of Pediatrics was the attempt by the Children's Bureau to assert supremacy (as the pediatricians viewed it) over its domain. When the Children's Bureau, in implementing the EMIC program, was viewed as "an active factor in the practice of medicine throughout the United States, dictatorially regulating fees and conditions of practice on a federal basis," the academy did not hesitate to withdraw its support from the Children's Bureau and to request that all its health activities be placed under the regulation of the Public Health Service, a bureau controlled by physicians. As it noted then: "No method of practice or change in practice can be successful without the cooperation of the physicians of America, for on them rather than an administrative bureau lies the task of furnishing medical care."[69] Some fifteen years later, the Children's Bureau was still viewed as a "virtual dynasty" exerting powerful influence upon the destiny of American children.[70]

If the profession, as exemplified by the statements of the presidents of the Academy of Pediatrics, was condemning the Children's Bureau for too much interference in the development of standards and control over services, congressmen were later to concur because the bureau was bureaucratically inflexible. Commenting on the fact that a Seattle Children and Youth Project approved in 1966 had not served a single child by mid-1968, Senator Warren Magnuson noted that the bureau required each project to have a dentist, a chief nurse with a master's degree, a nutritionist with a master's degree, and so on. Inflexible bureaucracy had prevented children from receiving needed care.[71] Whether this congruence of interests between the Academy of Pediatrics and Congress reflected the lobbying of the medical profession as a whole is hard to say. It is sufficient to note that the Children's Bureau was, in fact, dismembered. In 1969 its health program was moved to the Public Health Service. Its other functions of child welfare and child research were moved to the Office of Child Development in the Office of the Secretary of Health, Education, and Welfare, where they languished. In essence, the federal government had acceded to the academy's demand of twenty-five years earlier.[72]

The demise of the Children's Bureau resulted in the dissolution of any federal institutional center of responsibility for children.

The scattering of its programs and the submergence of the children's health program in other community health programs within the Public Health Service indicate the decline of a federal focus for responsibility for child health care. What had originally distinguished the child health programs was that they were service programs as well as regulatory and supervisory. The Public Health Service, as a whole, in acceding to the interests of the medical societies, had operated few direct service programs. Thus, child health was subsumed under an organization which was not interested in taking broad responsibility for child health. The pediatricians could expect no further competition here.

A second threat to the pediatricians' responsibility for child health has been health educators. Schools have traditionally been viewed as convenient places where child health care can be carried out. That few schools have undertaken comprehensive programs must be examined. First, among those engaged in administering school health programs, there has been over the years a conflict between school nurses employed by school boards, and school nurses employed by public health boards which are dominated by physicians.

Second, there has been a conflict between the private and the public sectors. Private physicians, including pediatricians, have been reluctant to allow children to receive examinations in school if this will take the children away from their offices. They have couched the argument in terms of promoting continuity of care. There may also be an economic argument. Nevertheless, school systems have responded by arranging their health care system so that the schools care only for those children for whom private physicians are not available either because of cost or because of geographic maldistribution. This policy is reflected in an Academy of Pediatrics' statement:

In communities where a large number of school children do not receive adequate health care, school health programs may need to include screening and preventive and some treatment services until better sources of care are developed. For the majority of children in the United States, such school medical services are not necessary and may be ineffective because they have a regular source of health care.[73]

Third, there is the distrust that arises both among physicians and parents about the ability of educators and their staff nurses to diagnose correctly the problems that children may have. This concern has taken the form of worries about misclassification, "labeling," and the prescription of medications for hyperactive children.[74]

On the whole, schools have approached the responsibility for child health cautiously. Given their responsibility for education and the criticism which they have received for failing in that field, their reluctance to take on another responsibility is not surprising. Several attempts have been made to promote greater health services in the schools, but these have been mainly in the form of experimental projects, funded by outside sources.[75] How much of this caution has been due to recognition of opposition from the private sector, and how much is due to the school boards' own lack of interest, is not entirely clear. What is evident is that pediatricians have not had much competition from schools in providing health services.

The third source of competition for pediatricians has come from other physicians. The conflict between pediatricians and other physicians in their responsibility for children has been a threat not so much in the realm of who should set standards, but where care should take place. Over the years, the pediatrician has gradually expanded his clientele. Traditionally, the pediatrician had limited his practice to children under fourteen, but by the mid-1960s he had expanded his practice to include adolescents.[76] Whether pediatricians should be the exclusive primary care and "medical home" providers for children is a question on which pediatricians have been divided. In 1970, the Academy of Pediatrics debated the issue of whether primary care of children should be in the hands of a family physician or pediatrician, but came to no conclusion.[77]

Jurisdictional disputes have broken out between family physicians and pediatricians.[78] Since it is unlikely that at any time during the past twenty years there has ever been a sufficient and evenly distributed supply of pediatricians to serve all children in the United States, it is evident that if a policy to provide a medical home for every child were established, some of those "homes" would have to be provided by nonpediatricians or even nonphysicians. Thus, this jurisdictional dispute as applied to medical homes may be more apparent than real.

Who Sets Standards for Care?
If pediatricians have felt their perceived responsibility for providing child health care to have often been threatened, they have had

a much clearer hand in setting standards for that care. In the early days of this century, the government was the main body applying some minimum guidelines to assure good health for children. The Children's Bureau's most popular best-seller was *Infant Care*, which, written in layman's language, gave parents basic information about care of their baby, including hygiene and nutrition.[79] More important, the Children's Bureau set standards by supporting research in nutrition, which resulted in publication of standards of nutritional needs for children on relief.[80] Even these actions were new to government, for in 1908, one concerned physician noted, "there was no preventive medicine in public health."[81] But within thirty years, preventive maternal and child health services were part of the accepted functions of local and state health and welfare agencies.[82] The Children's Bureau and the state and local agencies set standards mostly on the qualifications of personnel rather than on the minimum standards necessary to achieve child health, but the Bureau also continued to promote services which would benefit children. During World War II, the Children's Bureau gained a great deal of experience in setting standards for prenatal and hospital maternity care when it administered the EMIC program.[83] The development of reliable Phenylketonuria (PKU) screening was financed by the successors to the Children's Bureau, who also successfully advocated the mandatory adoption of this test by the states.

The government's major incursion into setting standards for care occurred when Congress passed PL 92-603 in 1972. This law required the establishment of nation-wide physician groups to form Professional Standards Review Organizations (PSROs) to review institutional care funded through the Social Security Act. Although review of ambulatory care was optional under the law, simply the fact that the government was formally mandating standard setting and monitoring the care rendered by physicians and institutions was a significant departure from earlier governmental policy.

Aside from government, the other major group to set standards for preventive child care was the pediatricians. Their involvement grew slowly out of the perception that the maintenance of basic child health and hygiene seemed an integral part of what a pediatrician could offer as part of his services. Thus, pediatric textbooks at the turn of the century devoted over 10 percent of their content to nutrition and feeding.[84] Preventive care in a broad sense did not make its way into these books until the 1930s, but the profession as a whole developed increasing concern for its role in carrying out preventive pediatric care. The textbooks themselves referred most often (and briefly) to child hygiene in their introductory chapters, but a 1934 handbook of pediatrics offered an entire section devoted to preventive measures.[85]

More often than not, the concern for prevention in pediatrics was found in rhetorical statements rather than in textbooks or journals. From 1930 to 1978, pediatric textbooks devoted only about 4 to 8 percent of their pages to discussions of prevention.[86] The American Pediatric Society during its first forty years devoted more than half of its annual presidential addresses to child hygiene, but only sixty-eight out of the 1,196 papers presented at its scientific sessions were concerned with prevention in its broadest interpretation.[87]

Nevertheless, the 1920s and 1930s saw the flourishing of the well-child conference throughout the United States. Pediatricians trained during this period learned and accepted that well-child care was a part of pediatric practice. Preventive health clinics were operated by state or local health agencies, using local physicians to carry out the basic examinations. States and localities provided training for physicians in how to carry out these examinations.[88]

The American Academy of Pediatrics, formed in 1930, was more socially oriented than its rival, the American Pediatric Society, or its parent group, the American Medical Association.[89] Through the use of committees, the academy gradually established itself as the spokesman for standards in child health care. Within thirty years, the academy had published standards for infectious diseases, for newborns in hospitals, for child health care, and for school health. Since these books were published in many editions and were mailed to all members of the academy—which by 1977 numbered over twenty thousand—they became widely known.[90]

The academy expanded its activities in 1971 by forming the Joint Committee on Quality Assurance (JCQA), which studied methods by which to assess the quality of pediatric ambulatory care. Using the Delphi method and through surveys, the JCQA developed a series of criteria for appropriate care, both preventive (including well-child visits) and curative.[91]

Researchers evaluating programs also established criteria and standards by which to assess the care rendered. The majority of these evaluators were pediatricians, but their criteria and standards, although perhaps influenced by the activities of the academy, were established independently.[92]

Finally, standards were also set by groups or individuals whose interests related to children or preventive health. The National Education Association in conjunction with the American Medical Association established standards for school health appraisals.[93] In anticipation of national health insurance, several organizations and individuals set out recommended schedules for preventive medical care. These groups were the American Public Health Association, the Association of Schools of Public Health, and the Fogarty International Center. All three groups had engaged in standard-setting exercises previously, but this appeared to be the first time that all three were involved in standard-setting for preventive care.[94]

Although pediatricians were dominant in setting standards, one must keep in mind as well that they cared for fewer than half of the children in the United States.[95] One may well ask why this group had been delegated the task of setting standards for all children. The fact is that it was not as if pediatricians had elbowed out others waiting to undertake the job. Quite the contrary, they were among the few who attempted to systematize the tasks of preventive health for children. Few, if any, other organizations had shown much interest in the matter until the question arose of what procedures should be paid for in a public health insurance program.

No other group has taken on for itself the responsibility for child health care. In its advocacy role, pediatrics differed from other medical speciality groups.[96] There were two evident reasons for pediatric involvement. The first was a pediatrician's compassion for his clients and the recognition that much of what must be done to raise a healthy child had to be done outside his own office. The second was the pediatrician's own economic interests. Of course, the balance between these two interests was not the same for any given pediatrician at any given time, and as one noted member of the profession pointed out: " . . . pediatricians' interests and children's interests are not always the same."[97] This left pediatricians in an uncomfortable position as child advocates, while their societies remained the sole groups willing to set standards for child health care.

What Are the Standards for Preventive Care?

Standards for child health care may be applied in matters of time, procedure, and place. The first has to do with the frequency of procedures, the second with the procedures themselves, and the third with the place appropriate for such procedures. We have already examined the place appropriate for procedures as part of the analysis of the unresolved debate on the responsibility for providing a child's medical home.

To discuss the frequency of procedures separately from the procedures themselves is not to say that they are independent of one another. The periodic health examination is a series of screening procedures carried out at one visit. At what time a particular procedure is carried out depends on whether that procedure is effective for preventing or detecting disease at that point in a person's life. In addition, the examination of children also includes counseling, whose benefits may be independent of screening benefits and may be more effectively carried out at points in a child's life other than those at which the screenings are appropriate.

The belief in the periodic health examination for children is strong, but the validity, efficacy, or necessary periodicity of most of the tests which make up that exam have not been established.[98] Two points should be made about these procedures. First, opinion has varied greatly over time, and between different groups at the same time. Second, there have been very many of these procedures. A review of the literature during the past ten years on screening procedures for child health turned up some seventy different types of screening tests, with eighteen topics or diseases accounting for about 60 percent of all those discussed.[99] In this section, I shall examine the consensus on three preventive care procedures, all of which affected the EPSDT program: immunization, which has in the past seemed to receive high consensus as to its validity; developmental assessment, about whose validity there has been low consensus in the medical profession; and the frequency of the periodic examination itself, which has been the focus of changing opinions.

Consensus on Immunization

Immunizations have long been believed to be the single most effective measure in preventing disease. The first vaccination against smallpox occurred in the late eighteenth century.[100] Early vaccination was undertaken as a form of individual protection against a disease, but it gradually became recognized that if all or even most persons in a community were immunized, this would produce a herd immunity which would be much more effective if it could be maintained through adulthood by booster shots.[101] During the 1920s and 1930s diphtheria, tetanus, and pertussis (whooping cough) immunizations were developed and used, although some were never subjected to strictly controlled field trials.[102]

By the 1960s poliomyelitis vaccines had been tested, debated, and finally used, with the Sabin oral live vaccine winning out over the Salk killed vaccine because of its ease of administration and its ability continually to produce antibodies. During the following ten years, immunizations were also developed for measles, mumps, and rubella (German measles). Rubella vaccination was introduced not to protect persons from the disease itself, but to protect babies *in utero* for whom their mother's infection with the disease could lead to blindness, deafness, or other congenital defects. Thus by 1975 the public had available immunizations for the major childhood diseases. Meanwhile, because the last case of smallpox in the United States occurred in 1949, because any future cases would occur only through importation, and because the risks of immunization had become greater than the risks of catching the disease, the Public Health Service in 1971 recommended the discontinuance of routine smallpox immunizations.

From earliest times, governments had recognized the effectiveness of immunization. By the mid-nineteenth century, smallpox vaccination was compulsory for infants in Great Britain. In the United States, although the vaccination was even encouraged by an act of Congress, it was never mandated for infants. Physicians, however, continued to recommend it,[103] and although not compulsory for infants, vaccination did become compulsory for school entrance in fifteen states and territories by 1915. Twenty-one other states allowed local jurisdictions to enact compulsory vaccination regulations.[104] As table 4 shows, the trend toward mandated immunizations accelerated after 1962.[105] By 1976, forty-five states required children to have certain immunizations before admission to school.[106]

Neither in England nor in the United States were these mandatory laws rigorously enforced, particularly as the perceived risk declined.[107] In the United States, the lack of enforcement can be ascribed partially to the recognition that much of the need for im-

Table 4 States mandating immunizations prior to school entry

	1915	1962	1969	1976
Number of States with Any Mandatory Immunization Legislation	15	19	27	45
By Disease				
Smallpox	15	19	24	1
Diphtheria	—	9	18	43
Tetanus	—	6	16	41
Pertussis	—	6	16	37
Polio	—	7	20	44
Measles	—	—	17	45
Rubella	—	—	—	38
Mumps	—	—	—	2

Sources:

1915: John J. Hanlon, *Principles of Public Health Administration* (St. Louis: C. V. Mosby, 1964), p. 554.

1962: U.S., Congress, House, Committee on Interstate and Foreign Commerce, *Hearings on H.R. 10541: Intensive Immunization Programs*, 87th Cong., 2d sess., 1962, p. 14.

1969: Charles L. Jackson, "State Laws on Compulsory Immunization in the United States," *Public Health Reports* 84 (September 1969): 794.

1977: National Immunization Work Group on Consent, *Report and Recommendations of the National Immunization Work Groups*, submitted to the Office of the Assistant Secretary for Health (McLean, Va.: JRB Associates, 1977), appendix A–1.

munization occurred before the children came to school, and partially to the fact that attempts to enforce the immunization law would lead to violation of the school attendance law. Given a choice, it was always the latter law which was enforced by school boards, despite the consistent findings that mandatory immunization programs were legal.[108] The immunization laws therefore served more as statements of social hopes rather than as protection for the community.

In addition to these governmental attempts to make immunization mandatory, other public and private bodies set standards. The American Public Health Association (APHA) systematized information for control of infectious diseases in 1917 when it published its first *Control of Communicable Diseases in Man*. Originally, its primary objective was to provide information about the control of epidemics. Gradually, as its many editions expanded, its emphasis began to center around the surveillance of disease.[109] However, the information it dispensed on immunization appeared only in the context of particular diseases. One had to read through the entire book (117 diseases in the 1965 edition) to find out which immunizations should normally be provided for children.

The work that became most referenced was the Academy of Pediatrics' (AAP's) "Red Book." First published in 1938 as the *Report of the Committee on Immunization Procedures*, it contained information about eighteen diseases in a slim eight pages. By 1977, its 18th edition with more than three hundred pages had established it as the authority on primary immunizations, schedules, types, and cautions. Nearly all pediatric textbooks referred to the Red Book or adopted its schedule for immunization recommendations.[110]

The federal government in 1946 had developed its own Communicable Disease Center, [111] later expanded and renamed Centers for Disease Control (CDC), and Congress gave this agency the task of implementing the Poliomyelitis Vaccine Assistance Act of 1955 and the Vaccine Assistance Act of 1962. When the latter was passed, the House Committee Report noted:

The threat of epidemics of these diseases can be avoided and therefore the continuing threat constitutes a totally unnecessary risk. . . .
   The benefit to the country will be freedom from threat of epidemics. Economically, the Nation will benefit by the preservation of the productive capacity of individuals who are now handicapped as a result of these diseases.[112]

Through continuing congressional authorizations the CDC expanded its assistance to the states for a long list of diseases including diphtheria, whooping cough, tetanus, measles, rubella, tuberculosis, and venereal diseases; it also promoted RH factor testing. Meanwhile, the Surgeon General had in 1964 appointed an Advisory Committee on Immunization Practice (ACIP) to assist the Public Health Service on the status of immunizing agents and their use.

For governmental agencies, the purpose of immunization policy was to reach masses of people in the shortest time possible with the fewest number of visits. Government was less concerned about the protection of individuals. Pediatricians, however, believed they could be more leisurely in scheduling immunizations for their patients.[113] Therefore, they recommended frequent return visits for immunizations. However, by 1977, visits for different immunizations tended to be combined, due to the felicitous finding that antibody production seemed to benefit from simultaneous administration of several vaccines.

Standards changed with time as new vaccines became available and as field trials demonstrated that the effectiveness of particular vaccines depended upon the time of their administration. Table 5 shows some of the changes in these recommendations for primary immunizations for children in the Red Book between 1955 and 1977. The Red Book stressed that the times established were recommendations and could be altered according to the needs of individuals, particularly if an individual were ill or if a particular disease were epidemic in the community. The Red Book schedule was intended to be a flexible guide for physicians, not a set of inviolate rules.[114]

The belief in both the effectiveness and the importance of immunizations continued to grow. These beliefs were reflected in statements from pediatric textbooks, such as: "Routine immunization is a standard part of the well child care delivered by most physicians."[115] If the effectiveness of immunization were actually a tenet of faith among physicians and the public, then one would expect the procedure to be carried out routinely. This was not the case. Immunizations were endorsed, but not enforced. In immunization, as in other recommended preventive child health procedures, a discrepancy existed between standards and practice.

Two sources illustrate this discrepancy. The first is the annual number of cases for any disease for which immunizations were available. Although the incidence rate of pertussis, tetanus, and diphtheria declined precipitously from 1952 to 1970, cases still persisted long after the vaccines were available.[116] For both polio and measles, the number of cases dropped off rapidly after introduction of the vaccines: polio after 1955 and measles after 1965. Nevertheless, cases persisted, indicating the absence of complete immunization of the population.

These findings are confirmed by annual immunization surveys. Immunization with full doses for polio, DTP (combined diphtheria-tetanus-pertussis), and measles together never reached more than 79 percent of children aged one to four. The proportion of children with immunizations remained fairly consistent over time, with the proportion who received no doses declining. However, the polio immunization rate, which was high following the postwar polio epidemics and the introduction of the vaccine, declined to 60 percent in the 1970s.[117]

The pattern was similar, although the rates were higher, for children five to nine years old. For this age group the proportion of

Table 5 Primary immunization recommended by the American Academy of Pediatrics, Report of the Committee on Infectious Diseases ("Red Book")

Interval	1955	1964	1966	1970	1977
1 mo.	DTP (1–2 mo.)				
2 mo.	DTP (2–3 mo.)	DTP OPV 1	DTP OPV 1	DTP TOPV	DTP TOPV
3 mo.	DTP (3–4 mo.)	DTP OPV 3	DTP OPV 3	DTP	
4 mo.		DTP OPV 2	DTP OPV 2	DTP TOPV	DTP TOPV
5 mo.	Smallpox				
6 mo.				TOPV	DTP (TOPV optional)
9 mo.		Measles	Tuberc. Test[a]		
12 mo.		Smallpox	Smallpox Measles	Measles Tuberc. Test	Tuberc. Test
15 mo.	DTP (16–18 mo.)	DTP OPV 1,2,3	DTP TOPV	DTP TOPV Smallpox	Measles Rubella Mumps
24 mo.		Tuberc. test	Tuberc. Test DTP (3 yr.)		DTP (18 mo.) TOPV (18 mo.)
4 yr.	DTP	DTP Tuberc. Test	Tuberc. Test	DTP (4–6 yr.) TOPV (4–6 yr.) Smallpox (4–6 yr.)	DTP (4–6 yr.) TOPV (4–6 yr.)
6 yr.		Smallpox Tuberc. Test	TD, TOPV Smallpox Tuberc. Test		
8 yr.		DTP	Tuberc. Test		
12 yr.		TD	TD Smallpox	TD Smallpox Mumps	Td (14–16 yr.)

Abbreviations:
DTP: Diphtheria and tetanus toxoids combined with pertussis vaccine
OPV: Oral polio vaccine
TOPV: Trivalent oral polio vaccine
TD: Combined tetanus and diphtheria toxoids
Td: Adult type combined tetanus and diphtheria toxoids.
[a]Tuberculin test recommended every year or half year for children likely to be exposed.

children with a full set of polio vaccinations declined from 91 to 77 percent between 1964 and 1975. The proportion of children with DTP immunizations remained between 80 and 85 percent. Although measles immunizations took some time to become used, by 1977 they were more frequent among both age groups (63 and 76 percent, respectively) than polio immunizations.[118]

Nonwhite, central city, and rural children were less likely to be appropriately immunized.[119] These were the same populations believed to have inadequate access to physicians. However, even in private practice, a study showed that among two-year old children who were "active" patients only 32 percent had completed their immunizations.[120] Those receiving care at public health clinics fared slightly better, with 49 percent immunized.[121] Although this failure in immunization practice was denounced by the pediatric profession,[122] its cause most often was laid at the door of the public or the parents.[123] Others viewed the problem as one of combined failure on the part of the public, health professionals, and government officials.[124] Whatever the case, the promulgated standards were not being implemented.

Childhood immunization illustrates a case where a consensus regarding intent was agreed upon with relatively little controversy.[125] Yet the standards promulgated for polio, measles, and DTP immunization, which had been in existence for more than fifteen years, had not been followed in practice by physicians, public health officials, or by the public at large. When new standards or vaccines were introduced, a certain amount of controversy existed; but in the cases of DTP, polio, and measles, the immunization programs which had become accepted and undebated by 1965 were still poorly carried out. One can well ask if consensus truly exists if those who endorse a program do not then carry it out.

Consensus on Developmental Assessment

Developmental assessment appeared as a recommended procedure in all three editions of the Academy of Pediatrics' *Standards for Child Health Care*. It also appeared frequently in pediatric textbooks. It is one of many screening procedures which make up the child health examination. It is also a screening measure that has had little consensus as to its efficacy or merit, but that nevertheless persists.

One of the difficulties in assessing the efficacy of developmental screening is that researchers and clinicians are not clear as to what they mean by developmental assessment. First is the issue of whether developmental assessment refers to all neurological, psychomotor, psychological, and emotional development, or only to some segment of them. "Developmental assessment" implies the inclusion of mental development along with physical development. One can assume that such an assessment includes screening for both mental retardation and mental health, but this distinction is rarely specified. A second issue arises from the confusion between developmental screening and developmental assessment. In Britain, the former has usually been taken to mean a quick screening test while the latter refers to more complete diagnosis of conditions which may follow from a positive result on a screening test.[126] However, in the United States, this distinction is often blurred, and the two words, screening and assessment, are used synonymously.

For a screening program to be effective, three sets of criteria must be met: the first relates to the disease, the second to the test, and the third to the economic, social, and personal costs engendered by the tests and the savings achieved by early detection of disease.[127] For efficacious treatment of a disease, one must first have a thorough knowledge of what the disease is, the course it will follow if left untreated, and the knowledge that treatment is effective and available. In the case of mental retardation, both the definition of the condition and its natural course may be known only through symptoms, and its course cannot be predicted or altered except in the case of some genetic defects. For mental disease or emotional problems, the definition may be more difficult, and the natural course is rarely known with any certainty. These mental and emotional problems are seemingly intractable to predictive screening.

Some of these problems are reflected in the fact that reliable figures of incidence and prevalence of these conditions are hard to find. The Joint Committee on the Mental Health of Children reported in 1970 that 2 percent of all children needed immediate psychiatric care, and that an additional 8 to 10 percent could be helped by mental health workers.[128] The number of mentally retarded children in 1970 was estimated at around 2.8 million, or about 3 percent of all children under twenty, with another 1.5 million mentally ill.[129] Two other authors, however, reported higher figures for both mental illness and mental retardation, which, taken together, reached 17 percent of the child population.[130] If the estimates of prevalence vary so widely, it is possibly because the disease is not clearly understood, and because its natural course is not easily followed.

Thus the diseases or conditions to be screened for in developmental assessment are not clear, their course is not clear, nor is the treatment that should be used for any disease clear. In fact, for some developmental conditions, the best attitude may be one of wait and see. The greatest danger is when a child is mislabeled—identified as having a problem when he does not—or when the problem is only of a transitory nature. In either of these cases, a child is treated as if he had a problem when he does not, creating unnecessary worry and perhaps more severe psychological disturbance.

The second criterion is that the test or tests used be simple, accurate, reliable, and acceptable. Although at least a dozen tests are commonly used, such as those employed by Kaiser-Permanente,[131] the major developmental test in the United States has been the Denver Developmental Screening Test (DDST). No other test in use has had its record of experience in testing in different situations and among different groups. Among other tests, it was recommended by the American Academy of Pediatrics[132] and specifically for use in the EPSDT program.[133] In 1976, thirty-three states reported that the test was used in their EPSDT programs.[134]

Critics noted three distinct drawbacks to the use of this test. First, it took too long (about fifteen to twenty minutes to fill out the test form). The response to this objection was to develop a shortened version which took only five minutes for a parent to fill out.[135]

Second, the DDST's rate of false positives was too high, thus forcing the rest of the health system to cope with many normal children who had been sent on unnecessarily for diagnosis when nothing was wrong with them, an inconvenience for the children and their parents, an unnecessary expense for the taxpayers.

The third drawback of the DDST was that it was considered to be ethnically and socially biased. The test tended to produce a higher frequency of questionable findings when it was performed on children of low socioeconomic status above two years of age.[136] Similar problems were noted in its use in England.[137] For this reason, many public programs and clinics with large minority populations among their clients tended not to use the DDST in their screening assessments.

After 1975, HEW encouraged several attempts to create better tests or guidelines for developmental assessment, particularly because the EPSDT program recommended such testing. The American Orthopsychiatric Association in its study stressed that no culture-free tests were available but needed to be developed.[138] Similar concerns were voiced by the American Association for Psychiatric Services for Children[139] and by the Children's Defense Fund.[140]

The implementation of the EPSDT program stimulated the need to develop appropriate instruments for assessing the mental development of children. After 1975, work accelerated to arrive at a validated, culture-free test. As of 1981, such a test does not exist. This means that developmental assessment cannot meet one of the major criteria for a screening program.

The third criterion for a screening program to be effective is that there must be consensus on the social and economic benefits of the procedure. It is here that developmental assessment was most vulnerable. The Children's Defense Fund concluded that because of the unreliability of the tests and the dangers of labeling, specific tests for developmental screening should not be used in the EPSDT program.[141] Instead, data should be gathered from the usual pediatric assessment and from conversation with the parents and observation of the child about a child's developmental milestones. Some consensus could be found on the need to discover children at risk for slow development, but this was tempered with the realization that good treatment was not always available and that the risks of misidentifying children also brought high costs.

This case of developmental assessment illustrates the problems of implementing a nation-wide screening program for poor children when the scientific community does not have agreed-upon criteria and standards for carrying out the program. Developmental assessment is just one of the many screening procedures. If it fares particularly badly in its test of efficacy, it is not far behind that of many other specific tests. For example, height and weight are routinely measured at every well-child visit, but no studies have shown that these measurements are useful in detecting unsuspected disease.[142] Others have asserted that there are few substantiated screening procedures in infancy and childhood,[143] and that the efficacy and effectiveness of primary care processes have not been established.[144] It is evident that there are honest differences of opinion about screening tests and their applicability.

Thus, the lack of consensus extends to nearly every procedure which makes up the well-child examination. This may account for the different reports received about what is actually carried out in the exam. If there is no consensus, then individual physicians are free to practice as they see best. However, this compounds the problems of policy makers who are asked to set minimum standards for health care for which the government will pay.

Consensus on the Frequency of the Well-Child Examination

The well-child examination has been discussed earlier in terms of its history, acceptability, and prominence in pediatric practice. Recommended frequency, which we will now examine, has varied over the years. Between 1930 and 1949, pediatric textbooks recommended an average of twenty-three visits for the first year of a child's life (table 6). These numerous visits were seemingly left over from the earlier weighing visits at milk stations and did not always involve full-scale care.[145] Exactly what services were to be provided was not always spelled out by the authors of the pediatric texts.

The major shift in recommended periodicity schedules took place after 1950, when the weekly weighings were discontinued. In recent years, the trend was toward less frequent visits during the first year of life (from 9.5 visits during the 1950s to 6.3 visits during the 1970s), and an increase in the number of visits during the second year of life (from 1.8 visits during the 1950s to 3.0 visits during the 1970s). One does not want to examine these findings too closely, since they are averages taken over many books with different authors, editions, and publication dates, but they do show a general trend toward fewer health examinations for children.

The American Academy of Pediatrics, which began publishing standards for child health care only in 1967, showed an even greater tendency to decrease recommended visits. In 1967, the academy recommended a child be seen from nine to twelve times during his first year (table 7). Five years later, the number of recommended visits had decreased to six to nine. Within another two years, a guide to screening prepared under contract to the Department of Health, Education, and Welfare recommended only five visits during the first year. This number was then reiterated in the

Table 6 Average number of recommended physician visits for each age group: Pediatric and preventive medicine text and reference books

Age	Years of Publication			
	1930–1949	1950–1959	1960–1969	1970–1978
0–11 months	22.5	9.5	9.0	6.3
12–23 months	7.5	1.8	2.9	3.0
24–35 months	7.0	1.8	1.7	1.6
36–71 months	11.0	3.2	2.7	2.7
6–14 years	40.5	8.0	6.2	8.9

Source: Appendix 2.

Table 7 Number of recommended screening visits for each age group: Academy of Pediatrics

Book	0–11 mo.	12–23 mo.	24–35 mo.	36–71 mo.	6–14 yr.
Standards of Child Health Care, 1967[a]	9–12	4	2	2	8
Standards of Child Health Care, 1972[b]	6–9	2–4	1	2	8
Guide to Screening for the EPSDT Program, 1974[c]	5	2	1	2	3
Standards of Child Health Care (for well children who receive competent parenting), 1977[d]	5	2	1	2	3

[a]Council on Pediatric Practice, *Standards of Child Health Care* (Evanston, Ill.: American Academy of Pediatrics, 1967), pp. 18–29.

[b]Committee on Standards of Child Health Care, *Standards of Child Health Care*, 2d ed. (Evanston, Ill.: American Academy of Pediatrics, 1972).

[c]William K. Frankenburg and A. Frederick North Jr., *A Guide to Screening for the Early and Periodic Screening, Diagnosis and Treatment Program (EPSDT) Under Medicaid* (Washington, D.C.: Social and Rehabilitation Service, Department of Health, Education, and Welfare, 1974), pp. 55–56, 63–64.

[d]Committee on Standards of Child Health Care, *Standards of Child Health Care*, 3d ed. (Evanston, Ill.: American Academy of Pediatrics, 1977), pp. 13–14.

1977 standards published by the academy. Thus, within a ten-year period the number of visits recommended for children during their first year had decreased by more than half. A similar trend occurred for the total number of recommended visits for children between the ages of six and fourteen years: they declined during that period from eight (one visit annually) to three visits for the whole period.

What accounts for this steady decline in the recommended number of visits? One can catch a glimpse of the debate as it unfolded in the pages of *Pediatrics*, the journal of the American Academy of Pediatrics. The worth of child health supervision was questioned with the observation by Alfred Yankauer that: "Unfortunately, consensus is weighted heavily by traditions of the past and ingrained customs of the present."[146] Those who argued against this position acknowledged that the idea of child health supervision may have been oversold, but that the well-child visit served as a point of entry to medical care for many sick children who would otherwise not receive it,[147] and it also functioned to teach and counsel as well as to detect disease.[148] This debate was then reflected in the academy's 1977 edition of *Standards of Child Health Care* which emphasized that its recommendations were only a guide for "those well children who receive competent parenting, and who are growing and developing satisfactorily."[149] This left those children at higher risk presumably in need of more frequent visits, but no guidelines were given. It is possible that the earlier, more frequent standards were established for those higher risk children, but if so, they were not applied that way. It is also possible that the standards had changed. Possibly both are true.

The shift to decreased recommended frequency of examinations occurred as well in the public health literature. As table 8 shows, the number of recommended visits steadily decreased, to a point even below that proposed by the academy. The rationale for these schedules were not often given with the schedules, but the pediatric literature did not provide much better guides, particularly since there have been few controlled trials of the efficacy of any particular schedule with any particular group of children. Although over time there had been little consensus on the *frequency* of necessary well-child visits, there was a consensus among pediatricians and public health officials in the late 1970s that ten to fourteen well-child visits altogether were appropriate for a child

Table 8 Recommended number of screening visits by age group: Assorted individuals and organizations, 1973–1977

Author	Infant[a] 0–1 yr.	Preschool 1–6 yrs.	School Child 6–16 yrs.	Adolescent 16–20 yrs.	Total 0–20 yrs.
Breslow, 1973[b]	4–6	1	1	1	7–9
American Public Health Association, 1974[c]	7	6	10	2	25
Fogarty Task Force, 1974[d]	5–7	8–10	2–3	2–3	17–23
Frankenburg and North, 1974[e]	5	5	3	1	14
Fogarty Task Force, 1976[f]	5	2	2	1	10
American Academy of Pediatrics, 1977[g]	5	5	3	1	14
Breslow and Somers, 1977[h]	5	2	3	1	11
HEW Working Schedule for CHAP Proposal, 1977[i]	4	4	3	1	12

[a]Visits recommended for the age of 12 months have been assigned to this category.

[b]Lester Breslow, "Incorporation of Preventive Medical Services in National Health Insurance," paper prepared for the Office of Management and Budget on Behalf of the Association of Schools of Public Health and the Association of Teachers of Preventive Medicine, 19 November 1973, in John E. Fogarty International Center, *Preventive Medicine, USA* (New York: Prodist, 1976), pp. 90–93.

[c]American Public Health Association, "Proposed Preventive Benefits to be Covered on a First Dollar Basis under National Health Insurance," 16 July 1974, in Fogarty Center, *Preventive Medicine, USA*, pp. 85–90.

[d]Fogarty International Center Task Force, "Preventive Medical Services for National Health Insurance," prepared under the auspices of the Office of the Assistant Secretary for Health, Department of Health, Education, and Welfare, May 1974, in Fogarty Center, *Preventive Medicine, USA*, pp. 93–101.

[e]William K. Frankenburg and A. Frederick North, *A Guide to Screening for the Early and Periodic Screening, Diagnosis and Treatment Program (EPSDT) under Medicaid* (Washington, D.C.: Social and Rehabilitation Service, Department of Health, Education, and Welfare, 1974), pp. 55–56, 63–64.

[f]Fogarty Center, *Preventive Medicine, USA*, pp. 39–43.

[g]Committee on Standards of Child Health Care, *Standards of Child Health Care*, 3rd ed. (Evanston, Ill.: American Academy of Pediatrics, 1977), pp.13–14.

[h]Lester Breslow and Anne R. Somers, "The Lifetime Health-Monitoring Program," *New England Journal of Medicine* 296 (March 1977): 602–603.

[i]U.S., Department of Health, Education, and Welfare, working draft for Child Health Assessment Program (CHAP), Susan Morgan, personal communication, 1978.

between birth and the age of twenty-one. The basis for this consensus remains elusive.

Moreover, as with immunization, a discrepancy remained between what seemed to be accepted in the medical profession (particularly the pediatric profession) and what was actually being practiced. Using a standard set by the academy, one study found that only one-third of infants from middle-class neighborhoods, and only one-twentieth of babies from the ghetto, received the recommended health supervision during their first year.[150] In another study of five-year olds in pediatricians' offices, only 12 percent had a recorded hemoglobin or hematocrit test, while only 20 percent had a recorded hearing test. Some of these tests may have been carried out without being recorded or the child may have received them outside the doctors' offices, but as the authors of the study pointed out, the most likely explanation was that "judgments about the advisability of some of the procedures varied among the practitioners. This appeared to be an individual rather than a group phenomenon. None of the practitioners rejected or accepted all of the procedures."[151]

This individuality of opinion was reflected by a pediatrician who said in 1967, when the academy published its first standards, that four examinations during a child's first year would uncover most defects, and who concluded that, for middle-income families, "we find it superfluous to see children for routine examinations except during the infancy period and for one pre-school examination."[152] The physicians at Kaiser-Permanente recommended pediatric multiphasic testing once every three to four years for children aged four to fourteen, while recognizing that they did not have data sufficient to suggest optimal ages or frequency for retesting.[153]

Is There Consensus?

The short answer to this question is "no." For children's immunizations, despite the consensus on standards which had been established by the Academy of Pediatrics in its publications, physicians were falling far short of providing these services to the children who were ostensibly under their care. For developmental assessment, the use of any measure had commanded so little consensus that one cannot even talk of a discrepancy between standards and practices. For the well-child exam, the consensus on frequency had been lacking for some time.

Pediatricians undertook very seriously their responsibility for setting standards. Yet one cannot but conclude that the standards which they developed over time were perhaps more needed by the profession than by children. Certainly, that proportion of the population which was receiving care at pediatricians' offices was not, for the most part, the poor; nor was it those identified as high-risk children. Thus, with the rise of social demands and programs of the 1960s, the standards which had been set for one group of children were demanded by others. The pressure of this demand should have caused the reexamination of the criteria for preventive pediatric care in the 1970s. However, for the middle-class child, seen by pediatricians, the general habit remained to recall infants frequently during the first year of life. It is perhaps not surprising that the standards set for those children under a pay-as-you-go system were reexamined only when they were to be applied to children for whom the government would pay.

What Do Policy-Makers Know and When Do They Know It?

Given the dissensus among pediatricians and other health professionals as to what the standards for preventive health services for children should be, it is not surprising that policy-makers have known very little about the scientific basis for their decisions affecting preventive health for children; and even when they have had information, they have often chosen to ignore it. If only a moderate consensus exists and most physicians do not act on it anyway, one should not expect legislators and agency administrators to weigh their views very heavily. To illustrate this point, in this chapter I shall examine two policy decisions relating to immunization, which, as we saw, had a fairly high consensus; and one relating to the frequency of well-child examinations under EPSDT, which had a fairly low consensus.

The Swine Flu Fiasco

In February 1976, a few cases of swine flu diagnosed among recruits at Fort Dix, New Jersey, became the basis for a series of presidential and congressional decisions leading to the flu immunization campaign of that year.[154] The program had been sold as a medical necessity: it was said that if the population of the United States were not immunized by the time of the winter flu season, it was probable that a serious epidemic of swine flu would break out. Since this was the virus which had caused the pandemic of 1918–1919 which had resulted in millions of deaths, concern was understandable. However, several questions needed to be answered: Would a swine flu epidemic break out? If an epidemic did break out, would it be as virulent as it had been in 1918–1919? Was it possible to develop the vaccine and vaccinate the American people before the next flu season set in? According to the Director of the Center for Disease Control of the Public Health Service, the answer to each of these questions was "yes."

The decision that President Ford made that April was based on an action memorandum presented to him by the Secretary of Health, Education, and Welfare, reflecting the best scientific information (culled mainly from the Center for Disease Control). Even at the time of his decision to proceed with the program, there was some disagreement within the scientific community as to whether such a program was necessary. As the summer months slipped by, and no further cases of swine flu appeared, more questions were raised within the scientific community about the value of the program.

The swine flu immunization program was difficult to implement. Although Congress, easily impressed by the danger of the flu epidemic, appropriated $130 million, the program required as well the development of vaccine in sufficient doses for a mass program. However, the drug companies were unwilling to manufacture the vaccine until they received insurance coverage to free them from liability for possible adverse effects of the vaccine. Congress and the president had been firmly convinced of the need for the immunization program by the scientific community. Therefore in August Congress voted for the insurance coverage, which then permitted the drug companies to begin manufacturing the vaccine.

By September there had still been no new verified cases of swine flu; but the vaccine was ready for distribution, a process which proved to be difficult, as most states did not have sufficient personnel and equipment to administer the doses. By November a few cases of swine flu had appeared, all except one, among people who handled pigs, and in all cases a mild disease from which the victims recovered uneventfully. The public had resisted the immunization campaign from the beginning, at first because it was not convinced of the seriousness of the problem, and eventually because serious side effects were emerging in a small proportion of those vaccinated. Because of these problems, and because no epidemic had shown itself, the Public Health Service finally suspended the immunization campaign in December 1976.

The program had been a fiasco. Some of the scientists had done such a good job of promoting the need for the program that at no time did they help policy-makers see that if an epidemic failed to appear, policy should perhaps be revised. However, the scientists, particularly at the Center for Disease Control, who had committed themselves and their institutions to the program, plunged on straight ahead despite cries from within the scientific community and despite increasing resistance from the American public in the late fall of 1976. The policy-makers—Congress and the president—would have been better off had they required that proponents of the program set up a schedule of retrenchment measures to be implemented if certain events, such as the projected epidemic, did not take place.

Policy, once set in motion, is difficult to stall. Had Congress been fully aware of the questions within the scientific community about the immunization program, or at least more skeptical of the scientific "facts," it could have saved a lot of money, or built a mechanism for retrenchment decisions. At the beginning, the program might have seemed politically useful to President Ford. An immunization effort would allow him to sponsor a major health program at a time when he had been cutting back on almost all existing health and social programs. Once implemented, its very visibility required perpetuation. Some of the scientists had sold a program which they could not have stopped even had they wanted to, because the program fitted the political needs of those whom they enlisted to support it. In American politics, for a short while, being against the flu immunization program became a bit like being against motherhood.

Thus politicians did not investigate because they liked the program for political reasons; and those scientists who had hitched their fortunes to the program were also reluctant to call for a reassessment. If policy-makers had wanted to know, they could have found out that there was serious question within the scientific community about continuing the program once no epidemic appeared. However, the politicians had as much to lose by stopping it midway as by continuing, particularly if the threat of epidemic were maintained. The detracking of a program once it has been set in motion is difficult unless the program turns out to have been a disaster. Fortunately, the disaster in the case of swine flu immunization was relatively small as disasters go. However, its failure left the public, the scientific community, and politicians strongly skeptical about mass immunization programs.

Making Immunizations Mandatory

In Connecticut in 1978, the headline of the *New Haven Register* read, "Doctors Disagree on Giving Shots for Rubella."[155] The previous day the Committee on Public Health and Safety of the state legislature had heard testimony on a law which would require certification of immunization for diphtheria, pertussis, tetanus, poliomyelitis, measles, and rubella for all children entering school.

Children who were not immunized would be excluded from school. Proponents of the bill included a representative from the Connecticut Medical Society, two epidemiologists from the state health department, and three local health directors. They cited the decline of cases of these diseases since immunizations had been available. They also cited the decline and disappearance of congenital rubella syndrome in newborn infants since the introduction of the rubella vaccination in Connecticut. They noted that the American Academy of Pediatrics, the Academy of Family Practice, the American Public Health Association, and the American Hospital Association all supported this immunization program.

However, it was the opponents of the rubella immunization who provided the longest and most emotional testimony. They argued that in the case of rubella it would be better for girls to acquire natural immunity which would be lifelong, rather than to have immunizations whose effects would wear off and might not be renewed. They also felt that pediatricians should have the right to make decisions about rubella immunizations for their own patients.[156] The opponents were two private-practice pediatricians from different towns of Connecticut, and an infectious disease epidemiologist from a local hospital. While the proponents noted that the majority of physicians and scientists recommended the rubella immunization, the opponents countered with the fact that the American Medical Association, the Center for Disease Control, the American Academy of Pediatrics, and the Public Health Service had also recommended the swine flu program, a comment designed to catch the ear of legislators who had all been aware of that program's failure.[157]

The Director of the Preventable Diseases Division of the State Health Department pointed out that all children did not have access to pediatricians, and he saw the matter as "an issue of a public health policy . . . in opposition to individual philosophy of patient care."[158] On the other hand, a pediatrician said:

What is at risk here . . . is whether I as a . . . physician will be coerced by the state and the Department of Health to do something I feel . . . may be a problem with my child later.[159]

These differing opinions had their effect on the legislators. As one expressed it:

I'm really in a quandary here, because I have the utmost respect for both of your testimonies. . . . How do I as a layman of the legislature decide this issue in the next fourteen days, so that I do not allow one child of the state to be hurt by my decision?[160]

The legislators, in their final decision, were most influenced by the opponents, who had provided the most effective testimony and with whom they had the closest political relations.[161] The bill, as drafted by the committee, allowed for exemptions from rubella immunization. That such exceptions might undermine a mandatory program was not considered. On a vote of seven to two, the committee then sent the bill to the full assembly, where it was passed into law.[162]

In both these immunization programs, the policy-makers made their decisions for political reasons. In the case of the swine flu program, the political rationale coincided with the majority scientific opinion at the time of the program's inception. In the rubella controversy, the legislators made their decision against the majority of scientific opinion. One may conclude that if scientific opinion is to have any practical effect, it had better coincide with political necessity.

The Frequency of Screening under EPSDT
The EPSDT program recommended to the states procedures for screening children. The guidelines, published in 1972, listed these procedures, but did not provide any guidance on the frequency of screening.[163] The states were therefore on their own for devising how many screening visits they were willing to pay for under Medicaid.

State standard-setting for frequency of screening resulted in an extraordinary assortment of patterns, which are shown in table 9. Between the ages of birth and twenty-one, one state (Wyoming) approved only three visits, while three states (Massachusetts, North Carolina, and Washington) approved twenty-five visits. The differences were just as great for children under six years old. For that age group alone the range was 1.67 (Wyoming) to fourteen visits (Connecticut); the median was six visits.

Even more surprising was the variety of patterns that developed. North Dakota approved screening every other year regardless of the child's age. Eight states approved payment for screening visits annually, also regardless of the child's age.[164] This annual pattern seemed to be regional: half of these states comprised all of

Table 9 Number of screenings paid for by state EPSDT programs, by age, 1977

State	Under 1 yr.	1–2 yrs.	2–3 yrs.	3–4 yrs.	4–5 yrs.	5–6 yrs.	Total Screenings, 0–6 yrs.	Total Screenings, 0–20 yrs.
Region I								
Connecticut	5	3	2	2	1	1	14	18
Maine	4	2	1	(1:2 yr.)[a]		(1:3 yr.)	8.33	13
Massachusetts	5	2	1	1	1	1	11	25
New Hampshire	5	2	1	1	1	1	11	15
Rhode Island	once every 18 months						4	12
Vermont	5	2	1	1	(1:3 yr.)		9.67	14
Region II								
New Jersey	1	1	1	1	1	1	6	12
New York	5	2	1	1	(1:2 yr.)		10	13
Region III								
Delaware	1	1	1	1	1	0	5	9
D.C.	2	1	1	1	0	0	5	10
Maryland	2	1	1	1	(1:2 yr.)		6	11
Pennsylvania	5	1	1	(1:2 yr.)		(1:3 yr.)	8.33	14
Virginia	5	3	2	1	(1:2 yr.)		11.5	17
West Virginia	4	2	1	1	1	1	10	16
Region IV								
Alabama	0	0	1	0	1	0	2	6
Florida	1	1	1	1	1	1	6	11
Georgia	3	1	1	0	1	0	6	9
Kentucky	1	1	1	1	1	1	6	21
Mississippi	1	1	1	1	1	1	6	7
North Carolina	4	2	1	1	1	1	10	25
Tennessee	(7:2 yr.)		1	1	1	1	11	12
Region V								
Illinois	4	2	1	1	1	1	10	15
Indiana	1	1	1	1	1	1	6	13
Michigan	2	1	(1:2 yr.)				5	8
Minnesota	2	3	1	(1:2 yr.)			7.5	11
Ohio	1	1	1	1	1	1	6	5[b]
Wisconsin	5	1	1	1	0	1	9	17
Region VI								
Arkansas	1	1	1	1	(1:3 yr.)		4.67	9
Louisiana	3	1	0	1	0	1	6	11
New Mexico	1	1	1	1	1	1	6	12
Oklahoma	1	1	1	1	1	1	6	21
Texas	1	1	1	1	1	1	6	21[c]
Region VII								
Iowa	1	1	1	1	1	1	6	21
Kansas	1	1	1	1	1	1	6	21
Missouri	1	1	1	1	1	1	6	21
Nebraska	1	1	1	1	1	1	6	21

Table 9 (continued)

State	Under 1 yr.	1–2 yrs.	2–3 yrs.	3–4 yrs.	4–5 yrs.	5–6 yrs.	Total Screenings, 0–6 yrs.	Total Screenings, 0–20 yrs.
Region VIII								
Colorado	5	3	2	1	1	1	12	18
Montana	1	1	1	1	1	1	6	21
North Dakota	(1:2 yr.)						3	11
South Dakota	4	2	0	1	1	1	9	13
Utah	1	1	1	1	1	1	6	11
Wyoming	1	0	0	0	(1:3 yr.)		1.67	3
Region IX								
Arizona	No Medicaid Program							
California	5	2	1	1	(1:2 yr.)		10	13
Hawaii	1	1	1	1	1	1	6	12
Nevada	3	1	(1:3 yr.)				5.33	9
Region X								
Alaska	5	2	1	1	1	1	11	19
Idaho	5	2	1	1	(1:2 yr.)		10	15
Oregon	3	1	1	0	1	(1:2 yr.)	6.5	14
Washington	4	1	1	1	1	1	9	25

Sources:

Screenings for children under 6: Community Health Foundation, "A Comparison of Periodicity Schedules and Screening Packages in 50 State EPSDT Programs with Head Start Health Requirements," Evanston, Ill., February 1979 (mimeographed).

Total screenings for children under 21: U.S., Department of Health, Education, and Welfare, "Comparison of EPSDT Program Costs for Present and Mandated Periodicity Schedules," Washington, D.C., HCFA, Office of Child Health, 7 December 1978 (mimeographed).

[a](1:2 yr.) means once every 2 years; (1:3 yr.) means once every 3 years.

[b]The discrepancy between the number of screenings under the age of 6 and the age of 21 result from the information being drawn from two different sources.

[c]Texas was shown as paying for only 11 visits in the HEW source, but interviews with Texas officials in 1978 indicated they would pay for up to 21 visits.

Region VII of the Department of Health, Education, and Welfare. These patterns are surprising in light of the recommendations which had been made during the previous ten years. A glance at tables 7 and 8 shows that all the recommendations had emphasized more frequent visits for very young children than for older children.

What accounts for this perplexing diversity of patterns? Since in most states the EPSDT program was administered by the welfare or social services departments, there were not many, if any, persons in those departments with the knowledge or expertise to plan such schedules. The Department of Health, Education, and Welfare therefore recommended to the states that they consult with their health departments, state pediatric societies, and other groups in drawing up their periodicity schedules. To assist the states, HEW commissioned the Academy of Pediatrics to write a guide to screening which was then distributed to the states.[165]

Connecticut is an example of a state whose Welfare Department not only consulted other groups in devising its schedule, but finally turned the job over to the Health Department. The Health Department was more than willing to work with the Welfare Department, and also consulted the state chapter of the Academy of Pediatrics. Since the Health Department was developing standards as well for all child health clinics in the state, the two tasks fell together.[166] The result was that the final periodicity schedule followed closely that of the academy.

Texas, on the other hand, introduced a program of annual screening. So firmly entrenched was this annual pattern that when the director of the EPSDT program was asked in 1978 why this pattern had been established, he said he assumed it was a federal decision.[167] In fact, in 1978 no one connected with the Texas program could answer how or why the annual schedule had been established. One person suggested that it had been set in 1974 by the former medical director of the Medicaid program. Another official suggested that the decision to screen annually was simply based on "administrative convenience." That is to say, it was supposed to be easier to find every child once a year or once every two years than, for example, to have to find some children four times a year and others not at all. Whatever the reason, no one responsible for the Texas EPSDT program could explain its periodicity schedule.

In 1977, the Department of Health, Education, and Welfare itself was charged with drawing up a recommended schedule of visits for children to be used in regulations for the proposed Child Health Assessment Program. One participant in the process said that they just sat around, looked at what everyone else was doing, and came up with an estimate which was limited only by the maximum number of visits they should allow between the ages of birth and twenty-one years. The proposed schedule turned out to be similar to that of the academy (see table 8).

One must conclude that there was probably a good deal of "administrative convenience" in the decisions taken by states, particularly by those with biennial or annual periodicity schedules. Another form of administrative or political convenience was to mandate, as Wyoming did, few screenings to keep the costs of the program low. Even if the consensus, as we have seen, was not perfect, there was nevertheless some consensus among pediatric groups. This consensus was ignored by many states whose policymakers could follow a course that fit more closely with their administrative or political needs.

The Technological Constraint

Pediatricians had succeeded in becoming the major arbiters of standards for child health, but they could not enforce these standards among other pediatricians or primary-care physicians, much less see that they were part of the standards of public programs. A good deal of the problem lay in the fact that the standards, although not capricious, were not backed up by well-conducted statistical studies. There were no tests that showed whether or not following these standards would result in maximum health at minimum cost. There had been too many visits for well middle-class children, and perhaps too few for the seemingly well poor children. Moreover, the demand for a medical home raised questions about whether the purpose of these standards was to provide the best comprehensive care or to fill the physicians' offices. Logically, it seemed absurd for a child to go to several different health care providers for his care, and several studies indicated that satisfaction and care were better in comprehensive care settings. Nevertheless, it was not clear that the medical home needed to be a physician's office or even a clinic. If pushing children to physicians' offices were seen as even part of the goal, however, then the standard-setting exercise may well have been a case where children's interests and pediatricians' interests did not coincide.

Politicians, used to acting politically themselves, tend to see other groups as acting politically as well. Thus, the pediatrician's move toward responsibility for standard-setting may have been viewed in the political arena as not entirely disinterested. What had been termed a debate revolving around the best medical interests of the child was, in fact, a debate as to whose interests were best served. It came down to the old fight between private and public medical interests. Yet this debate was never explicitly stated. Neuhauser observed the effects of this kind of debate on legislators when optometrists and ophthalmologists squared off against one another in Massachusetts:

Put yourself in the position of a state legislator. All day long you are talking to the truckers who want the tolls lowered, to the unions about closed shop, to the racetrack owners, the liquor store owner, on and on. Each group is wrapping up its narrow economic interests in motherhood and the flag. Then the eye doctors come in trading insults. What is the legislator to think, other than that these people are like all the rest, fighting over who will get the nickel?[168]

In pediatrics, the debate was more subtle, and occurred mainly in the national arena. Legislators and administrators, called upon to determine how often and by whom children should be seen (at least when their care was paid for out of public funds), were hard-pressed to evaluate the validity of claims for frequent well-child examinations. Nor could they assess the value of the doctor's office versus public clinics, or "comprehensive care" providers versus public "mass screening" clinics. Not all private physicians were "comprehensive care providers," and not all public clinics were "mass screening clinics." Nor did either label of "comprehensive care" or "mass screening" have much to do with the quality of care rendered at these places.

The problem of standards for preventive health care for children could be viewed as the continuing philosophical struggle between the adherents of Hygeia and Aesculapius. In fact, a more practical struggle was taking place among people with special interests. The result was that no clear medical or scientific consensus existed for the technologies used in the EPSDT program. Screening and periodic health examinations for children did not have the solid backing of the scientific community. The dissensus among health professionals, reflected in their practices, indicates that no clear technology existed which could be implemented by policy-makers in their programs. In this environment, policy-makers could set their own standards. However, when they did, the EPSDT program became vulnerable to attack from public and professionals alike because it mandated either excessive or insufficient care. With uncertainty as to what the appropriate standards were, it proved difficult to judge what the program should or should not do. Nor did it endear EPSDT to state bureaucrats and legislators concerned with rising costs. A program of uncertain scientific validity was hard to defend. Thus the technological constraint, hypothesized in the introduction, did exist for the EPSDT program. Whether scientific dissensus is necessarily fatal to a program is hard to say from this one case. Other social programs with unclear goals, such as Head Start and the poverty programs, have survived, and EPSDT survived, too, if a bit lamely.

Conclusion: Politics, Prevention, and Policy

The incorruptible observer must hold that the Command, if it had seriously desired it, could have overcome those difficulties which prevented a system of continuous construction. There remains, therefore, nothing but the conclusion that the Command deliberately chose the system of piecemeal construction. But the piecemeal construction was only a makeshift and therefore inexpedient. Remains the conclusion that the Command willed something inexpedient.—Strange conclusion!

Franz Kafka, *The Great Wall of China*

The EPSDT program was born in ambiguity and uncertainty. Considering the bureaucratic and congressional neglect discussed in part I, the institutional constraints of part II, and the technological constraint of part III, it is all the more surprising that the program functioned as well as it did. Children who earlier had not had care did get screened and treated, even if not necessarily counted. State agencies managed to set up networks of screening services. As did Texas, some states successfully constructed case management systems. Nationally, in 1978, nearly two million out of 10.2 million children eligible for Medicaid had been screened and most of them who needed treatment had received it. Why the program functioned at all is the reverse side of the picture I have been painting, and is worth a comment here. First, although state administrators may have objected to the increased service and administrative costs associated with the program, they were not philosophically opposed to the provision of preventive health services for children. Second, welfare rights organizations and other child advocates lobbied successfully for the program and, where lobbying failed, they filed suits which were, for the most part, successful. Finally, because some physicians in some states were already providing the equivalent of EPSDT services to some Medicaid-eligible children, the program requirements were not always all that novel.

Certainly the most instrumental part of the program goals, to screen needy children, had been met by the program. EPSDT had been less successful in organizing a system of preventive and curative services for poor children, that is, in meeting those goals that would directly improve children's health. Even those states which achieved a high level of screening services often failed to integrate the provision of health services. Moreover, many states did not even accomplish the screening of children, much less the concomitant follow-up and treatment. State legislatures were unwilling to invest sufficient funds in the program to carry it out; states resisted federal attempts to apply penalties; states had trouble finding screening and treatment providers. Sometimes, no implementation would have occurred without legal suits brought on behalf of the welfare recipients.

These and other conclusions must be tempered by the recognition that reliable data on the program were hard to obtain. The federal government, particularly in the early years, never seriously invested resources in routine reporting and evaluation, and when it did, evaluations usually took the form of demonstration projects which had special dispensations and therefore were not informative about how the program would work under less than hothouse conditions. Thus after more than eight years of implementation, the federal government still had only very limited research on which to evaluate the program. The studies which are yet to be done should evaluate the effect of the EPSDT program on the health of children. Such studies take time and cannot be expected within six months or a year, because effects would not likely appear so quickly. That neither federal nor state governments seriously invested in the evaluation of the program may indicate that they had only limited interest in the effect of the program on child health, or that they accepted uncritically the premise that screening would lead to better health and that there was no need to evaluate a program whose benefits were self-evident.

The question remains: Why did this well-intentioned program go awry? There seems to be three major reasons. First, the EPSDT program was an attempt to introduce on a mass basis a new technology whose value had never been tested. Mass screening for specific ailments had been introduced in the 1940s and 1950s, but the mass physical examination, although popular, and highly promoted by the medical profession, had never been seriously evaluated for efficacy. When it was, results were mixed, at best. For children, the standards which had been recommended in pediatric textbooks had been tried among middle-class children, but the extent to which they were actually applied even to them was unknown. Among no groups of children had mass screening techniques ever been tested for efficacy in randomized clinical trials.

One can argue that EPSDT was basically bad policy. What it set out to do could not be done with the technology proposed and available. It set out to prevent unnecessary crippling and deaths among children; it proposed to accomplish this by a system of screening, a technology that was accepted but whose worth was unproved. Like the Oakland Project, where the economic philosophy behind the program was inadequate, the medical philosophy behind EPSDT was faulty. Pressman and Wildavsky showed how the unemployment program in Oakland used means, such as loans to the Port of Oakland, that could not achieve the stated goal of relieving unemployment. The EPSDT program had similar problems. If the goal were to prevent unnecessary crippling and death among children, the most effective program was not necessarily the one chosen—secondary prevention, or screening—which could for the most part detect diseases only after they arose. A more effective program might have mandated primary prevention. Or, if the goal were to provide comprehensive care, a more effective program might have been to pay particular providers on a capitation basis for all necessary health care for the child.

The assumption was that the technology of screening was effective in preventing disease. This technology, however, was untested; there was no consensus among professionals as to the minimum standards which were appropriate for child health care. The standards which had been set for middle-class children were not suitable, and had perhaps been set as much in the interests of the pediatricians as of children. These observations have the advantage of hindsight. The framers of the 1966 HEW *Program Analysis*, who proposed the screening program, had no way of knowing that screening was not efficacious since to that time there had been little testing. Nor could they predict that during the next ten years the scientific consensus behind screening would evaporate. The problem for the EPSDT program was not that health professionals disagreed, but that everyone assumed that they agreed.

As the public in the 1970s became more and more impatient over conflicting claims, consensus in the scientific community became a matter of increasing concern. The National Institutes of Health formalized the need to achieve scientific consensus by holding consensus conferences on specific controversial subjects and then having a panel of experts come to a consensus. On many occasions this was successful and the recommendations of the panel were adopted as policy by the federal government and by individual physicians.[1] If there were true conflict, however—as there was, for example, in a cervical cancer screening conference, where the consensus panel ended with a split vote[2]—then public confidence in the opinion of the scientific community necessarily decreased. If the scientific community cannot agree, it seems unreasonable to expect the lay public or policy-makers to come down firmly on one side or the other. Moreover, no consensus conferences were held at all on the standards for preventive child health care.

The discovery that scientists disagree on the merits of a procedure where it has been assumed they agree constitutes a serious constraint on a program. Given differences of opinion among scientists, policy-makers may choose to accept the dominant scientific opinion—as they did in the case of the swine flu immunization program. Or they may choose to accept a minority scientific opinion if that group has good political access to them and the decision makes political sense—as the committee of the Connecticut State Legislature did in the case of rubella vaccination. Finally, they may choose what is administratively expedient—as did those states which chose annual health exams for children under the EPSDT program.

The lack of consensus among medical and scientific professionals is a persistent problem. Scientists may honestly differ. It is frustrating for policy-makers to find programs such as immunizations or periodic health examinations thrust on them as scientifically and medically correct only to learn some years later that this is not so. When new evidence appears, this opinion shift is understandable, indeed necessary. However, programs are often promoted far beyond their scientific merits. Scientists should take these facts to heart and recognize that if they set standards or engage in policy-making on questionable scientific grounds, they may jeopardize the credibility of the entire scientific community. More importantly, in the case of EPSDT, they jeopardized a program of health services to poor children by allowing questions to be raised about the validity and efficacy of the technology used.

The lessons for the political community are that scientists and physicians have interests just like everyone else and that those interests influence their policy recommendations. This truism should not need to be stated were it not for the fact that the scientific community, particularly health professionals, lose sight of it and advance all sorts of unvalidated claims about what health programs will accomplish. The "War on Cancer" is a recent and well-known example.

In the long run, this technological constraint may be intractable. Its existence, however, should serve notice to scientists and physicians not to introduce new programs in public policy until they are more firmly grounded scientifically, or introduce them with straightforward admission of uncertainty—the most honest but politically most difficult course.

The second reason the EPSDT program went awry was because the strategy of the framers was to base the program on existing institutions as they found them. Thus EPSDT was thrust into a political environment which seriously hampered its implementation. In the same way that the EPSDT program was required to use technological means (screening) inappropriate to the goals (preventing and treating potentially handicapping conditions), the administrative means of working through the then-existing institutions and programs were also inappropriate. If, as the program advocates came to suggest, the EPSDT program was designed to bring comprehensive health care to every child eligible for Medicaid, then the means of working through the federal-state system, and relying on the bureaucratic capacity of state health and welfare agencies, was inappropriate, particularly since the actual means were merely to establish a method of paying providers, not to build up the institutions to administer such a program.

That the welfare agencies in the two states studied had ideologies which were similar and which emphasized the efficiency and growth of the agency should have been an asset to program implementation. In both states, however, the agencies were ill-considered by their respective state legislatures and although they commanded vast resources in the state budgets (up to one-fourth of state funds), they were constantly having to battle for the additional resources needed for EPSDT.

The EPSDT program framers presupposed that health agencies would provide considerable help. However, health agencies in both Texas and Connecticut had been engaged in devolving their power on local agencies; in Connecticut, at least, this policy was so successful that by the mid-1970s, the department was practically out of the business of providing health services and had lost power and resources needed to manage public health. In Texas, the health agency set up a special screening unit for its EPSDT contract, but it isolated this unit from the rest of the health department and from the rest of the health care delivery system. This led to a highly fragmented delivery system which offered offense to no one, particularly not to private physicians and the Texas Medical Association, but which provided inadequate services to poor children.

The ideologies of health and welfare agencies have been little explored in the literature. The present study suggests that the ideology of the health agencies was most inappropriate for administering or even subcontracting for services for the EPSDT program. The health agencies, as constituted, were not ideologically adequate to the task of assisting EPSDT implementation. However, without further studies of such ideologies, it is difficult to know whether the pattern discerned in the two states is typical of state health and welfare agencies across the country.

The fact that states initially lacked the bureaucratic capacity to carry out the EPSDT program was not an overwhelming constraint. Texas managed to overcome this constraint and put together a credible case management system, reaching large numbers of children. Its program was extremely costly, and it seemed likely that the state would not maintain such an effort over an extended period of time if the federal pressure to implement were lessened. A federal policy to purchase such capacity for the states would have considerably advanced the program, particularly in states such as Connecticut which lacked the capacity for case finding and MMIS.

Federal inability to achieve the goals of the EPSDT program in the states resembled the weaknesses of the new towns in-town projects. As in the program studied by Derthick, EPSDT exceeded the limits of effective decentralization and pushed into the realm of programmatic disorder, where the center could neither compel compliance nor inspire creative solutions to implementation dilemmas.

The EPSDT experience also suggests some ways to overcome this problem on the assumption that local autonomy is not necessary in health programs of this type. States strongly resisted EPSDT and particularly the penalty provision. Most of state resistance had to do with the costs which the program would engender for them. To carry out the program properly would require information systems and staff; it would raise costs of payments to medical providers for the newly-discovered eligible children, and raise costs for the treatment of their newly-discovered conditions and ailments. At least in the short run, such a program could not but cost the states money. The coercion of compliance procedures and penalty sanctions could not work as long as the federal government considered the program a matter of federal-state cooperation. Cooperative federalism did not work in this case. If the federal government wanted such policies carried out, it would have to go much farther to overcome state resistance. This would mean buying state cooperation. Whether this means a matching rate of 90 to 100 percent is not entirely clear, but the matching rates which the federal government offered and continued to offer even in the CHAP revisions were not sufficient to overcome this strong state resistance. To achieve implementation of a program of this complexity, the federal government would have to exercise its economic power (as it did with Medicare and Social Security) by financing and running the program on its own and allowing time for the growth of bureaucratic capacity.

This solution is deceptively simple. If the federal government were to pay whatever necessary to buy state "cooperation," the institutional constraints, at least those discussed, would wither away. However, such a solution presupposes that the goal of achieving health services for poor children takes precedence over state autonomy. Although it has long been a popular notion among conservatives that more responsibility should be devolved upon the states, these findings suggest that any programs embodying such proposals will, when not desired by the states, run into much the same implementation problems as EPSDT: lack of state willingness to participate, health agency inability to mobilize resources, and lack of bureaucratic capacity. Such programs are unlikely to survive—which may be what the conservatives intended. State social welfare goals must be seen as necessarily more restricted than federal ones for two reasons: because states are parochial in interest, limited to concerns within their own borders (and perhaps not even that); and because their means of raising funds to support these activities are constrained by regressive tax systems. Thus, giving responsibility to the states is likely to result in fewer and less well run social programs—scarcely a recipe for successful social policy during periods of high inflation and unemployment.

One constraint not hypothesized at the outset of this study, but which emerged during analysis, was the effect which a lack of facilities and resources had on the development of the EPSDT program. Simply stated, the absence of providers of health services, whether because they refused to participate or because they simply did not exist in sufficient numbers in all parts of the United States, hindered implementation of the law. Paying for services was not sufficient if there was no one to provide them. This constraint relates directly to three others: ideologies, the absence of case management systems, and the lack of a scientific consensus on goals for maintenance of health. Administrative capacity and institutional strength were all the more important because the states were dealing with a fragmented provider system. The consensus problem reflects the fact that if physicians do not agree with the local or national standards, they will not abide by them.

The dearth and maldistribution of physicians helped determine the organization of the EPSDT program. Texas chose to operate its EPSDT program as a closed system, allowing access to screening only through special health department clinics and mobile units, and requiring that diagnosis and treatment be handled only by the private sector. While this produced a manageable program and succeeded admirably in providing screening services to a large number of eligible children, such a system fragmented health services and in that way made it difficult for poor children to receive the care they needed.

Connecticut, on the other hand, working through the open system, was unable to manage or monitor the program, or to provide services to large numbers of children. Although children could be served in the regular mixed system of provider services, the state did not have the capacity to monitor such care, nor to see that it took place for the children whom the system did not ordinarily serve.

These findings about existing institutional structures reveal a fundamental policy dilemma. Either the federal and state governments can set up their own closed systems which provide good screening services, but may fragment care; or they can operate within the open system, recognizing that they will have little or no control over the delivery of services so long as they function at their present level of competence. One solution to this dilemma is for state agencies to develop their bureaucratic capacity, but this is a protracted and expensive task.

Earlier, I noted that the ideology of welfare agencies did not seem to affect the implementation of EPSDT; that in the states of

Connecticut and Texas, with similar welfare ideologies, implementation was very different. This is not to say that ideology may make no difference at all, merely that welfare ideology made no difference to the implementation of EPSDT. Health agency ideology may, however, have influenced the shape of the program.

In the two states studied, the ideologies of the health departments were similar, with both agencies exhibiting a desire to withdraw from the provision of direct services and both state agencies being sensitive to the concerns of the state medical societies. Texas's fragmented EPSDT delivery system, which provided screening but not even the simplest or most elementary treatment, was designed not to offend private physicians and the Texas Medical Association. Such an attitude might make sense if the private sector were then to pick up all the care for all children in the state, but there was evidence that many parts of the state lacked health providers for diagnosis and treatment. The desire to be inoffensive to the private sector had resulted in second class services for the poor children who could least afford it. In Connecticut, the fragmentation also existed because many physicians were not willing to participate in Medicaid. Thus the open system of Connecticut was partially closed to those children who needed help.

It may be that compromising with the medical profession is a political necessity; but if so, and if the experience of these two states holds true elsewhere, the United States is doomed to halfway health programs that cannot be properly administered by the agencies to which they are assigned. In the case of EPSDT in Texas and Connecticut, these were the welfare agencies, but it is likely that the health agencies would have had no greater capacity nor would their ideologies have suited them well for taking on the requisite tasks.

The third reason for EPSDT going awry was its planners' and framers' incrementalist philosophy. The EPSDT program grew out of extensive work in the Department of Health, Education, and Welfare in 1966, but it received little attention from Congress when it was legislated, and not much more from HEW after it was enacted. So little attention did the program receive that it was dubbed a program without policy.[3] At least in its early years, an EPSDT policy was hard to discern and, as time passed, the policy in HEW and Congress wavered. Variance in federal directives allowed for variance in state performance. Thus the failure here is not one like that of new towns in-town or Oakland, where grandiose federal schemes are proposed but fail at the local level. It is a case in which modest, ambiguous plans fail at both the federal and state levels. If overambition were a fault for some federal projects, underambition seems to be as serious a fault in others.

EPSDT is a prime example of incrementalist philosophy applied to policy decisions and how such a policy may fail to accomplish program goals. The early planners were unclear about how the program should be implemented; they were even unclear whether the Crippled Children's Program or Medicaid should carry it out; and Congress failed to allocate sufficient funds to implement it. The estimates of what the screening component of the program would cost were always minimized in budget presentations to both the Office of Management and Budget and Congress. It was believed that the program could be carried out if the legislation were passed without drawing sufficient attention to the program to draw congressional scrutiny. The result was a program ignored, but also underfunded, which managed to survive by being discreet; this is scarcely a recipe for success. Moreover, the program was also subject to decrementalism after the CHAP amendments had failed in two Congresses and a Republician administration had taken office. By mid-1981, states were again receiving signals from the federal executive branch that the penalty would not be enforced and they could therefore again relax their programs. Although the decrementalism was still incipient, it was sufficient to illustrate the old adage that those who live by increments shall die by them. With neither an institutional base nor strong support from legislatures, EPSDT entered the 1980s as a highly vulnerable program. What makes this sad is that it was a program designed to care precisely for those most vulnerable in American society, poor and needy children.

Incrementalism is not always a hazard to programs. With just such a philosophy, the Social Security program of 1935 remained relatively immune from political tinkering and expanded enormously during the next forty years.[4] That such a strategy was not successful for EPSDT may be because the framers and advocates underestimated the limits of the institutions on which they were building their program. As it turned out, the task environment for the program was, as Lustick calls it, "non-decomposable."[5] To implement EPSDT required changes in many interested institutions and policies: to tinker with one, you had to tinker with the others. Provider participation depended upon payment which was tied to the state legislature, but it also depended upon the distribution of providers over which the states had little control. Client participation depended upon case management systems in state health or welfare departments which in turn depended upon state capacity and interest. The federal government had little control over any of these elements, and found it could not work on one piece of the system without working on the others. Because of the non-decomposability of the task, the incrementalist strategy may have been less effective than a more centralized approach. Thus, poor children were used as a flying wedge to restructure American health services and provide the basis for a national health insurance system. Since they and their parents lacked the power to command continued attention to their needs, EPSDT proved to be a frustration for its advocates and implementors. This finding suggests that equity in health care for poor children may best be achieved not by a piecemeal approach focusing on their particular needs, but by a program serving every person regardless of need or age.

The incrementalist strategy may have been a hazard to the EPSDT program for another, more important reason: it was established without any statement of principle. Politicians may have to choose short-term gains achieved through compromise and incrementalism at the expense of long-term gains of principle. For a politician, short-term gains are of greatest interest. His constituents acknowledge them immediately. There is no virtue in being known forty years hence as the person who enacted "X," because by that time, both the politician and his constituents will be long since gone. The strategy of incrementalism may be a political necessity for politicians, but this does not necessarily make it a virtue. Except for the 1966 HEW *Program Analysis* and President Johnson's 1967 message in which he sent the EPSDT legislation to Congress (quoted at the head of the introduction), there was no statement of principle involved in the EPSDT program. Perhaps politicians were afraid to say that what they were doing was extending the notion of equity in health services to poor and needy children. By not stating the principle, politicians were able to avoid the consequences of their actions. Bureaucrats charged with implementation had no such privilege.

Because there was no statement of principle for EPSDT, implementation was constantly constrained by values of competing groups as to what national policy should be. Physicians preferred to practice as they pleased without interference from health and welfare agencies; states preferred to administer without federal interference; the scientific community preferred to advocate standards of uncertain merit; state legislatures preferred not to spend money.

Thus, the question became one of whose values would prevail. Without a clear statement of principle from Congress, many values did prevail, but not the principle that any child, regardless of his means, should have equal access to health services.

The EPSDT program challenged the administrative and organizational ability of state health and welfare agencies to provide health care for needy children. Moreover, it challenged the medical and scientific community to explain clearly what minimum care was needed to promote good health among children. More than fourteen years after the program was enacted and nine years into implementation, politicians, administrators, and health professionals were still far from meeting that challenge.

The EPSDT program offers important lessons for any attempt to develop national health insurance in the United States. Like EPSDT, most national insurance proposals would rely on the present open system of health services, merely allocating to government the responsibility for paying the providers. As presently constituted, no state or federal agency appears to have the capacity to monitor care under such an open system. That there is little or no monitoring of care may not be a problem for most persons who are quite capable of managing their care themselves, particularly if they receive assistance in paying for it. It is, however, a severe problem for those very persons for whom the state becomes most responsible: the poor and the needy and the dependent. The children to be served by EPSDT were all from this group. Their needs could not be met by the open system, even when payment was available, because the providers did not exist, or would not accept them as clients, or because the children could not physically get to the providers' offices. The remedy we saw in Connecticut of making payment available for services was insufficient to provide care for those children. Texas's solution to set up a separate closed system was unsatisfactory because of the fragmentation it engendered.

Medicaid and EPSDT were enacted on the assumption that they would not change the then-existing modes of delivering health care. This philosophy underlay state reluctance to get involved in setting up systems which might actually have delivered more and better health care to poor children. EPSDT showed that providing states with additional resources to purchase preventive and curative care was insufficient without providing them with the resources to establish a delivery mechanism. One cannot buy into a system which does not exist. The same lesson would apply to national health insurance.

Any responsible proposal for a national health insurance system which seeks to serve the poor and the bewildered as well as the more advantaged must deal with the structure and organization of medical services, not just their financing. Government must either provide services directly, or have the power to organize others to do so. If the states are to perform either role, the federal government must somehow provide them with sufficient resources and incentives to act. Alternatively, the federal government can bypass the states either by directly employing health providers itself, or more indirectly by forcing changes in the way the open system operates. Many studies have already shown that the poor do not receive health care without government assistance. This study of EPSDT strongly argues that government assistance will not suffice unless the structure of American medical care itself is changed.

Appendix 1
Events Relating to EPSDT Penalty Regulations and Enforcement, and to the Proposed CHAP, 1972–1980

Regulations	Penalty Enforcement	CHAP Legislation
1972		
Fall: Congress enacts penalty of 1% to be applied to AFDC funds for failure to implement EPSDT in forming and service provisions		
1973		
Oct. 11: Proposed regulations signed by SRS Commissioner Dwight		
Dec. 19: Proposed regulations published; few comments received		
1974		
Spring & Summer: *National Journal* articles and TV program criticizing EPSDT's implementation	July 1: Penalty in effect according to law	
Aug. 2: Regulations published, Guidelines published (PRG–32) stating other compliance procedures remain in effect	Aug. 9,13,16: Conferences with state Medicaid directors to review new penalty procedures	
	Nov.: Penalty Reports due from Regional Offices on 1st quarter FY 1975; most are filed on time	
1975		
	May 12: General Counsel reports on penalties	
	June 2: Penalties announced for Pa., Ind., Minn., Mont., N.D., N.M., Hawaii	
Aug. 20: Proposed regula-	June 30: Calif. penalty an-	

Regulations	Penalty Enforcement	CHAP Legislation
tions published; over 100 comments received	nounced for 1st quarter FY 1975	
	Oct. 8: N.Y. penalty announced for 1st quarter FY 1975, making a total of $5.8 million in penalties	
	Fall: All 9 states request reconsideration	
1976 Spring: Penalty repeal under debate in HEW	Jan. 12: Pa. cited for 2nd quarter FY 1975	
	Feb. 20: HEW requires penalty reviews only every other quarter for states previously in compliance	
	July 7: Hawaii cited for 2nd quarter FY 1975	Nov.–Dec.: Discussions on amendments for EPSDT begin in lower levels of HEW
1977 Jan. 18: HEW Secretary Matthews refuses to sign new proposed regulations before he leaves office; suggests his successor refuse to sign as well	Jan.: General Counsel, reversing earlier opinion, says regulations cannot be retroactive and are nonenforceable because of vagueness	Jan.: Work begins in earnest on CHAP, proposed match dropped from 90% to 75%; total costs from $250 to $180 million
Feb.: National Governors' Conference asks for repeal of fiscal sanctions	By April: Additional penalties for 2nd quarter FY 1975 announced for Calif., Ind., N.M., N.Y., for a total of $12 million	Feb. 16: President Carter announces major child health initiative
		April 25: CHAP announced; legislation sent to Congress becomes H.R. 6706, S. 1392, in which penalty costs applied to administrative funds. Cost containment bill sent simultaneously
		Spring: Lobbying for CHAP led by Children's Defense Fund begins and maintained for next four years.
July: New proposed regulations awaiting signature of new HCFA director	July: HEW essentially stops penalty monitoring	July: CHAP receives lowest priority in House Health Subcommittee
Sept. 7: New proposed		Sept. 7–8: House Subcom-

Regulations	Penalty Enforcement	CHAP Legislation
regulations published; over 100 comments received		mittee holds hearings on CHAP
1978 March 9: HCFA requests hold on new regulations to await more state input	March 9: HEW announces to regional medical directors the suspension of penalty reviews	Feb.: Initial mark-up in Subcommittee on House CHAP bill provides for repeal of AFDC penalty retroactive to enforcement
		July 26: House Committee reports out CHAP
Sept. 20: Children's Defense Fund writes to HEW to request action on regulations		Aug.: Senate hearings on CHAP
		End Oct.: CHAP dies at end of 95th Cong. without having been voted on by full House or Senate
1979		
		Spring: Administration CHAP bills introduced to House and Senate; other versions introduced by Reps. Maguire and Waxman. Bills include retroactive repeal of penalty and new penalty applied to administrative funds tied to minimum performance standards
May 18: Final penalty regulations published		May: Child advocates lobby to make sure funds for CHAP are in 1980 budget
		June 7,11: House Subcommittee Hearings
		June 25: Senate Subcommittee Hearings
		July: Sen. Long puts a hold on CHAP in Committee
Oct. 1: New penalty regulations are effective	Fall: States petition HEW for suspension of penalty. HEW waivers, but after much advocacy lobbying	Oct.: House Committee reports out CHAP as H. R. 4962
		Dec. 11: House passes

Regulations	Penalty Enforcement	CHAP Legislation
	finally launches trial monitoring of regulations	CHAP tacking on many amendments including one requiring Congressional approval of regulations and anti-abortion provisions
1980		
		Spring: Presidential budget for 1981 requests $403 million for CHAP
	July: Penalty monitoring begins	April: House budget committee recommends only $40 million, assuming CHAP start will be delayed
		Dec.: CHAP, never reported out of Senate, dies with end of 96th Congress

Appendix 2
Pediatrics Textbooks, Reference and Practice Books, and Preventive Medicine Books

| Book[a] | Year of Publication | Active Prevention,[b] Percentage of Pages | Periodic Exam Recommended Visits | | | | | | Immunization |
			Schedule Source	1 Yr. 0-11 Mo.	1–2 Yr. 12–23 Mo.	2–3 Yr. 24–35 Mo.	3–5 Yr. 36–71 Mo.	6 Yr. & Over	Schedule Source
Pediatric Textbooks									
Holt and McIntosh, eds. *Holt's Diseases of Infancy and Childhood*, 10th ed.	1933	.9	not given	38	12	12	12–24	6 or 12 yearly	not given
Holt and McIntosh, *Holt's Pediatrics*, 12th ed.†	1953	1.6	ND[c]	ND	ND	ND	ND	ND	not given
Holt, McIntosh, and Barnett, *Pediatrics*, 13th ed.†	1962	2.4	ND	ND	ND	ND	ND	ND	not given
Barnett, *Pediatrics*, 14th ed.†	1968	1.1	AAP Red Book:[d] 1965[e]	3	2	0	1	1, then every 6 years	AAP Red Book: 1965[e]
Barnett and Einhorn, *Pediatrics*, 15th ed.†	1972	1.0	AAP Standards of Child Health Care:[f] 1967	9–12 but noted as every 4–6 wk. for 0–6 mo.; 2 per mo. for 7–11 mo.	4	2	3–6	1, then yearly	AAP Red Book: 1971
Rudolph, *Pediatrics*, 16th ed.†	1977	2.1	AAP Standards of Child Health Care:[g] 1972	7	4	2	2	1, then yearly	AAP Red Book: 1974

Book[a]	Year of Publication	Active Prevention,[b] Percentage of Pages	Periodic Exam Recommended Visits						Immunization Schedule Source
			Schedule Source	1 Yr. 0-11 Mo.	1–2 Yr. 12–23 Mo.	2–3 Yr. 24–35 Mo.	3–5 Yr. 36–71 Mo.	6 Yr. & Over	
Davison, *The Compleat Pediatrician*.	1934	8.0	not given	7	3	2	4	2, then yearly	not given
Davison and Levinthal, *The Compleat Pediatrician*, 8th ed.†	1961	18.0	not given	18	4	2	4	2, then yearly	AAP Red Book: 1955
Arena, *Davison's Compleat Pediatrician*, 9th ed.†	1969	1.8	not given	not given	not given	not given	not given	not given	AAP Red Book: 1969[h]
Nelson, *Textbook of Pediatrics*, 5th ed.	1950	2.4	not given	infant in nursery each day	not given	not given	not given	not given	AAP Red Book: 1943:[i] Pa. Dept. of Health[j]
Vaughan and McKay, eds., *Nelson Textbook of Pediatrics*, 10th ed.[k]†	1975	2.0	AAP: not given[l]	8	4	1–2	2–4	yearly	AAP Red Book: 1974
			not given	6	3	2	2	not given	
			AAP: not given[l]	not given	not given	not given	every 2 yrs. for school children		
Green and Richmond, *Pediatric Diagnosis*	1954	14.0	not given	12	not given	not given	not given	yearly	Batson & Christie: 1954[m]
Green and Richmond, *Pediatric Diagnosis 2*, 2d ed.†	1962	10.0	not given	not given	not given	not given	not given	yearly	AAP Red Book: 1961
Silver, Kempe, and Bruyn, *Handbook of Pediatrics*	1955	.05	ND	ND	ND	ND	ND	ND	AAP Red Book: not given
Silver, Kempe, and Bruyn, *Handbook of Pediatrics*, 12th ed.†	1977	4.0	Frankenburg	6	2	1	2	1 1 at 8–10	not given

Book[a]	Year of Publication	Active Prevention,[b] Percentage of Pages	Periodic Exam Recommended Visits						Immunization Schedule Source
			Schedule Source	1 Yr. 0-11 Mo.	1-2 Yr. 12-23 Mo.	2-3 Yr. 24-35 Mo.	3-5 Yr. 36-71 Mo.	6 Yr. & Over	
Silver cont.			and North: 1974[n]					1 at 11–12 1 at 13–15 1 at 16–21	
Harper, *Preventive Pediatrics: Child Health and Development*	1962	17.8	not given	8	2–3	2–3	2–3	2–3 at 6	AAP Red Book: 1961 (with polio modification)
Gellis and Kagan, *Current Pediatric Therapy 3*, 3d ed	1968	.8	not given	not given	not given	not given	not given	not given	not given
Gellis and Kagan, *Current Pediatric Therapy 8*, 8th ed.†	1978	.7	ND	ND	ND	ND	ND	ND	not given
Green and Haggerty, *Ambulatory Pediatrics*	1968	24.9	not given	7	4	3	not given	not given	AAP Red Book: 1966
Green and Haggerty, *Ambulatory Pediatrics II*, 2d ed.†	1977	10.9	AAP: not given	9	4	2	2	1, then yearly	AAP Red Book: 1974
Barness, *Manual of Pediatric Diagnosis*, 4th ed.	1972	1.2	not given	not given	not given	not given	not given	not given	ND
Forfar and Arneil, *Textbook of Pediatrics*	1973	2.3	not given	3	2	1	1 at 3, 1 at 4, not given at 5	not given	not given
Wasserman and Slobody, *Survey of Clinical Pediatrics*, 6th ed.	1974	1.1	not given	month-ly 1st 6 mo.; less freq.	3	2	4	2 at 6, then semi-annual	AAP Red Book: not given

| Book[a] | Year of Publication | Active Prevention,[b] Percentage of Pages | Periodic Exam Recommended Visits ||||||| Immunization Schedule Source |
			Schedule Source	1 Yr. 0-11 Mo.	1–2 Yr. 12–23 Mo.	2–3 Yr. 24–35 Mo.	3–5 Yr. 36–71 Mo.	6 Yr. & Over	
Wasserman cont.				next 6 mo.					
Shirkey, *Pediatric Therapy*, 5th ed.	1975	.3	not given	8–12	"Numerous" over next 5 to 6 yrs.				AAP Red Book: 1974
Ziai, *Pediatrics*, 2d ed.	1975	2.3	not given	12	not given	not given	not given	not given	AAP Red Book: 1973[o]
Pediatric Reference Books									
McKendry and Bailey, *The Infant and Pre-Schooler: Pediatric Problems in Family Practice*	1974	17.2	not given	5	3	1	yearly	yearly	Canadian Schedule:[p] 1970
Illingworth, *The Development of the Infant and Young Child Normal and Abnormal*, 6th ed.	1975	0	ND	ND	ND	ND	ND	ND	ND
Illingworth, *The Normal Child: Some Problems of the Early Years and Treatment*, 6th ed.	1975	5.5	ND	ND	ND	ND	ND	ND	Dept. of Health & Soc. Sec., England: 1972[q]
Hull, *Recent Advances in Paediatrics*, 5th ed.	1976	9.0	ND	ND	ND	ND	ND	ND	AAP Red Book: 1974; Dept. of Health & Soc. Sec., England[q]
Rendle-Short, *The Child: A Guide for the Paediatric Team*, 2d ed.	1977	4.0	not given	3	1	not given	1 at 3, 1 at school entry	not given	not given

Book[a]	Year of Publication	Active Prevention,[b] Percentage of Pages	Periodic Exam Recommended Visits						Immunization Schedule Source
			Schedule Source	1 Yr. 0-11 Mo.	1–2 Yr. 12–23 Mo.	2–3 Yr. 24–35 Mo.	3–5 Yr. 36–71 Mo.	6 Yr. & Over	
Rendle-Short cont.			not given	2	1	not given	not given	1	
Smith, *Introduction to Clinical Pediatrics*, 2d ed.	1977	3.8	not given	not given	not given	not given	not given	not given	AAP Red Book: 1974
Pediatric Practice Books									
Thompson and Seagle, *The Management of Pediatric Practice, A Philosophy and Guide*	1961	4.1	not given	not given	not given	not given	not given	not given	ND
Oberst, *Practical Guidance for Office Pediatric and Adolescent Practice*	1973	27.1	not given	5	4	1	yearly	yearly	not given
Bass and Wolfson, *The Style and Management of a Pediatric Practice*	1977	8.3	not given	in hospital and 1st month visit	not given	not given	not given	not given	AAP Red Book: not given (with modifications)
Preventive Medicine Books									
Leavell and Clark, *Textbook of Preventive Medicine*	1953	17.6	not given	12	2	2	2 at 4 1 at 5	yearly	not given
			La. State Univ. Pediatrics Service	2	every 6 months after 12-month visit; no cut-off year given				
Leavell and Clark, *Textbook of Preventive Medicine*, 3rd ed.†	1965	8.2	not given	8	2	every 6 months after 12-month visit; no cut-off year given			AAP Red Book: "up-to-date"
			not given	12	2	2	2 at 4 1 at 5	yearly	
Hilleboe & Larimore, *Preventive Medicine*	1959	3.2	not given	7	1–2	1–2	2–4	not given	not given

Book[a]	Year of Publication	Active Prevention,[b] Percentage of Pages	Periodic Exam Recommended Visits						Immunization Schedule Source
			Schedule Source	1 Yr. 0-11 Mo.	1–2 Yr. 12–23 Mo.	2–3 Yr. 24–35 Mo.	3–5 Yr. 36–71 Mo.	6 Yr. & Over	
Hilleboe and Larimore, *Preventive Medicine*, 2d ed.†	1965	3.8	not given	7	1–2	1–2	2–4	not given	not given
Clark and MacMahon, *Preventive Medicine*	1967	4.7	not given	10	4	yearly	yearly	yearly	AAP Red Book: 1966
Sartwell, ed., *Preventive Medicine and Public Health*	1973	2.8	not given	not given	not given	not given	not given	not given	AAP Red Book: 1970

[a]See bibliography for complete citation of all books. A dagger † indicates a new edition of the work cited in the preceding entry, or a work based on the preceding one.

[b]Active preventive care is defined as any action-oriented procedure by the medical care profession directed toward the maintenance of health. These procedures include: immunization, well-child visits, screening tests, school health programs, and counseling for parents. General discussions of growth and development, nutrition, or other health care issues were not defined as active preventive care.

[c]Not discussed.

[d]The AAP Red Book, often cited for appropriate years, is: American Academy of Pediatrics, *Report of the Committee on the Control of Infectious Diseases* (Evanston, Ill.: American Academy of Pediatrics).

[e]Although the author cites the 1965 edition, the AAP Red Book was not published in an edition for that year.

[f]Council on Pediatrics Practice, *Standards of Child Health Care* (Evanston, Ill.: American Academy of Pediatrics, 1967).

[g]American Academy of Pediatrics, *Committee on Standards of Child Health Care*, 2d ed. (Evanston, Ill.: American Academy of Pediatrics, 1972).

[h]Although the author cites the 1969 edition, the AAP Red Book was not published in an edition for that year.

[i]American Academy of Pediatrics, *Committee on Therapeutic Procedures for Acute Infectious Diseases and on Biologicals; Report* (Evanston, Ill.: American Academy of Pediatrics, 1943).

[j]"Adapted by Aims C. McGuinness from Procedures Recommended for the Pennsylvania Department of Health." No further citation is given.

[k]When books have different periodicity schedules reported in different places, all are listed.

[l]The American Academy of Pediatrics is cited but not the particular book or year.

[m]Blair Batson and Amos Christie, *Pediatric Clinics of North America* 1 (May 1954): 349–365.

[n]William K. Frankenburg and A. Frederick North, *A Guide to Screening for the Early and Periodic Screening, Diagnosis and Treatment Program (EPSDT) under Medicaid* (Washington, D.C.: Social and Rehabilitation Service, Department of Health, Education, and Welfare, 1974).

[o]Although the author cites the 1973 edition, the AAP Red Book was not published in an edition for that year.

[p]*Immunization and Related Procedures in Infants and Children*, prepared by the Infectious Service, The Hospital for Sick Children, Toronto, 1970.

[q]Department of Health and Social Security, *Immunization Against Infectious Disease*, prepared by Health Departments of Great Britain and Central Office of Information (London: HMSO, 1972).

Appendix 3
Persons Interviewed

Department of Health, Education, and Welfare, Washington, D.C.

Health Care Financing Administration (HCFA), formerly Medical Services Administration (MSA)

Keith Weikel, Commissioner, Medical Services Administration (MSA), 27 September 1977

Eugene Rubel, Special Assistant to Director, 28 September 1977

Galen Powers, General Counsel, 28 September 1977

Wesley Amend, Division of Information Systems, 27 September 1977

Robert Nakamoto, Acting Director, Division of Information Systems, 10 January 1978

Else Tytla, M.D., Consultant, 27 September 1977

Henrietta Duvall, National Center for Social Statistics, 9 September 1977

Annie Mayfield, National Center for Social Statistics, 9 September 1977

William Hickman, Research Director, MSA, 9 September 1977, 14 March 1978

Carl Allen, Office of Planning, MSA, 14 March 1978

Samuel Martz, Assistant Administrator for Financial Management, 10 January 1978

Beatrice Moore, Director, Office of Child Health, 27 September 1977, 14 March 1978

James Kolb, Deputy Director, Office of Child Health, 27 September 1977

Chapin Wilson, Program Monitoring, Office of Child Health, 28 September 1977, 10 January 1978

Office of the Secretary

Charles Lowe, M.D., Office of Child Health, 27 September 1977

Louise Liang, M.D., 10 January 1978

George Greenberg, Office of Planning and Evaluation, 1 November 1977, 10 January 1978

Bureau of Community Health Services, Office of Human Resources

Ralph Pardee, Deputy Director for MCHS Programs, 3 November 1977

John Schwab, Deputy Director for Child/Adolescent Primary Care, 3 November 1977

Connecticut

Estelle Siker, M.D., Director of Community Health, Health Department, 1 February 1978

Angela Sargent, Public Health Nursing Consultant, Health Department, 1 February 1978

Stephen Press, Director, Health Services, Department of Social Services, 30 March 1978

Stephen Locke, Consultant, Management Information Systems, Department of Social Services, 12 December 1977, 21 March 1978

Harold McIntosh, Program Director, EPSDT, Department of Social Services, 12 December 1977, 30 March 1978

Brian McCarthy, Research and Statistics, Department of Social Services, 21 March 1978

Stefanie Cameron, Office of Legislative Research, Legislature, 21 March 1978

Texas

Department of Human Resources, Austin

John Townsend, Assistant Commissioner for Coordination, 23 February 1978

Marlin Johnston, Associate Commissioner for Administration, 23 February 1978

Jean Shoemaker, Administrator, Medical Studies Task Force, 24 February 1978

Bob Smith, Program Manager, Medical Services Specialties, 21, 24 February 1978

Jack Eshelman, Medical Services Specialties, 21, 24 February 1978

Ray Kruger, former EPSDT Program Manager, 21, 24, 25 February 1978

Judy Krouse, Case Supervisor, 21 February 1978

Charlene Chunk Cavett, Case Work Supervisor, 22 February 1978

David Cook, Medical Data, 23 February 1978

Health Department, Austin

Hal L. Harle, M.D., Division Director, EPSDT, 22 February 1978

Dorothy Casey, Nursing Director, EPSDT, 23 February 1978

David Gray, D.D.S., Director Title XIX Dental Programs, 23 February 1978

Elizabeth Friend, Title XIX Medical Screening Clinic, 22 February 1978

James Drake, Immunization Program Manager, 24 February 1978

Health Science Center at San Antonio, University of Texas

Harold Dickson, Director, 20 February 1978

Arthur E. Britt, Assistant Deputy Director, 20 February 1978

Harry Meyer, 20 February 1978

Others

ZerNona Black, Director, Health Incorporated, San Antonio, Texas, 20 February 1978

Robert Dawson, EPSDT Outreach Supervisor, Health Incorporated, San Antonio, Texas, 20 February 1978

Bob Ramirez, EPSDT Project Director, Inman Christian Center, San Antonio, Texas, 20 February 1978

David Warner, Associate Professor of Public Affairs, LBJ School, University of Texas, 21, 25 February 1978

Wendy Lazarus, Children's Defense Fund, Washington, D.C., 9 September 1977

Judith Weitz, Children's Defense Fund, Washington, D.C., 3 November 1977, 13 March 1978

Donna Brown, Coalition for Children and Youth, Washington, D.C., 8 September 1977, 14 March 1978

Notes

Introduction

1. PL 90-248, sec. 302(a).

2. U.S. Department of Health, Education, and Welfare, *Data on the Medicaid Program: Eligibility/Services/Expenditures, 1979 Edition (Revised)*, Medicaid/Medicare Management Institute, Health Care Financing Administration, 1979, p. 53; and U.S. Department of Health, Education, and Welfare, Health Care Financing Administration, Office of Child Health (1977), unpublished table. Total costs for screening and treatment were estimated variously between $125 to $200 million.

3. U.S. Comptroller General, *Improvements Needed to Speed Implementation of Medicaid's Early and Periodic Screening, Diagnosis, and Treatment Program* (Washington, D.C.: General Accounting Office, 1975).

4. U.S. Congress, House, Subcommittee on Oversight and Investigations of the Committee on Interstate and Foreign Commerce, *Report: Department of Health, Education, and Welfare's Administration of Health Programs: Shortchanging Children*, 94th Cong., 2d sess., September 1976, p. iii.

5. Abraham B. Bergman, "The Menace of Mass Screening" (editorial), *American Journal of Public Health* 67 (June 1977): 601.

6. George A. Silver, *Child Health: America's Future* (Germantown, Md.: Aspen, 1978), p. 94.

7. Marian Wright Edelman, press conference, 22 June 1977. Mrs. Edelman was director of the Children's Defense Fund.

8. By 1978, health maintenance organizations in the United States had an enrollment of 7.3 million persons. *Group Health News*, December 1978, p. 10. In contrast, the Medicaid program served that same year 21.8 million persons. HEW, *Data on the Medicaid Program: 1979 Edition (Revised)*, p. 33.

9. Examples of these studies are: Karen Davis and Cathy Schoen, *Health and the War on Poverty: A Ten-Year Appraisal* (Washington, D.C.: The Brookings Institution, 1978); Martha Derthick, *New Towns In-Town* (Washington, D.C.: The Urban Institute, 1972); Charles M. Haar, *Between the Idea and the Reality: A Study in the Origin, Fate and Legacy of the Model Cities Program* (Boston: Little, Brown and Co., 1975); Daniel P. Moynihan, *Maximum Feasible Misunderstanding* (New York: Free Press, 1969); Jeffrey L. Pressman and Aaron B. Wildavsky, *Implementation: How Great Expectations in Washington are Dashed in Oakland; Or Why It's Amazing that Federal Programs Work at All, This Being a Saga of the Economic Development Administration as Told by Two Sympathetic Observers Who Seek to Build Morals on a Foundation of Ruined Hopes* (Berkeley: University of California Press, 1973); Gilbert Steiner, *The State of Welfare* (Washington, D.C.: The Brookings Institution, 1971); and also Eli Ginzberg and Robert M. Solow, eds., *The Great Society: Lessons for the Future* (New York: Basic Books, 1974), particularly Anthony Downs, "The Successes and Failures of Federal Housing Policy," pp. 124–45.

10. Erwin C. Hargrove distinguishes between evaluation research, which measures the achievement of an end product and implementation research, which has no such requirement. Its purpose is "to be able to say in an objective way that

strategy x will likely achieve consequences y with implications for goal z. . . . But it is the responsibility of the implementation researcher to explicate the trade-offs between a variety of program strategies. . . ." *The Missing Link: The Study of the Implementation of Social Policy* (Washington, D.C.: Urban Institute, 1975), p. 107.

11. See Lawrence M. Mead, *Institutional Analysis: An Approach to Implementation Problems in Medicaid* (Washington, D.C.: Urban Institute, 1977), esp. chap. I.

12. Charles E. Lindblom, "The Science of Muddling Through," *Public Administration Review* 29 (Spring 1959): 79–88; and Lindblom, *The Intelligence of Democracy* (New York: The Free Press, 1965), particularly chap. 9.

13. Graham T. Allison, "Conceptual Models and the Cuban Missile Crisis," *American Political Science Review* 63 (September 1969): 707.

14. David R. Mayhew, *Congress: The Electoral Connection* (New Haven: Yale University Press, 1974).

15. Lindblom, *The Intelligence of Democracy*, p. 277.

16. Jerome T. Murphy, *Grease the Squeaky Wheel: A Report on the Implementation of Title V of the Elementary and Secondary Education Act of 1965, Grants to Strengthen State Departments of Education* (Cambridge, Mass.: Center for Educational Policy Research, Harvard Graduate School of Education, 1973).

17. Pressman and Wildavsky, *Implementation*.

18. Derthick, *New Towns In-Town*.

19. Harvey Sapolsky, *The Polaris System Development: Bureaucratic and Programmatic Success in Government* (Cambridge, Mass.: Harvard University Press, 1972).

20. Murphy, *Grease the Squeaky Wheel*, p. 199.

21. Sapolsky, *The Polaris System Development*, p. 241.

22. *Ibid.*

23. See, for example, the analysis of President Jimmy Carter's difficulties in trying to apply engineering approaches to solve problems for which there are no objective solutions in William Pfaff, "Mr. Carter's Slide Rule," *New York Times*, 22 June 1979, p. A27.

24. *The Compact Edition of the Oxford English Dictionary* (Oxford: Oxford University Press, 1971), p. 2294. This dictionary cites Sir Thomas Browne with the earliest documented use of the word (1646): "Physicke is either curative or preventive."

25. See Hugh R. Leavell and E. Gurney Clark, eds., *Preventive Medicine*, 3d ed. (New York: McGraw-Hill, 1965), pp. 19–29; and also John E. Fogarty International Center and the American College of Preventive Medicine, *Preventive Medicine USA* (New York: Prodist, 1976), particularly the volume entitled *Theory, Practice and Application of Prevention in Personal Health Services*, pp. 2–3.

26. Harold D. Lasswell, *Politics: Who Gets What, When, How* (New York: P. Smith, 1959).

27. Eugene Bardach, *The Implementation Game: What Happens After a Bill Becomes a Law* (Cambridge, Mass.: The MIT Press, 1977), pp. 37, 42.

28. For a list of persons interviewed for this study, see appendix 3.

29. A description of the methods used is given in Anne-Marie Foltz, "The Politics of Prevention: Child Health under Medicaid" (Ph.D. dissertation, Yale University, 1980), appendix C.

Part I

Chapter 1

1. Edward R. Schlesinger, "The Sheppard-Towner Era: A Prototype Case Study in Federal-State Relations," *American Journal of Public Health* 57 (June 1967): 1034.

2. Willy De Geyndt, "Organization and Delivery of Comprehensive Health Services with Major Emphasis on Services to Children and on the Role of the Federal Government" (Ph.D. dissertation, University of Minnesota, 1970), pp. 40–41.

3. Schlesinger, "The Sheppard-Towner Era," pp. 1034, 1037. By 1935, however, states were sufficiently hungry that questions of constitutionality did not arise when even these three holdouts accepted the Public Assistance and Title V programs.

4. *Ibid.*, p. 1037.

5. The federal government had devised the strategy of requiring one state agency to supervise particular grants in order to reduce administrative chaos. For a discussion of the development of single-state agencies and their advantages and disadvantages, see Harold Seidman, *Politics, Position, and Power: The Dynamics of Federal Organization*, 2d ed. (New York: Oxford University Press, 1975), pp. 166–70.

6. A. L. Van Horn, "Crippled Children," *Social Work Year Book, 1947* (New York: Russell Sage Foundation, 1947), p. 139. For one of the most extensive studies to identify crippled children in New York, see Vernon Lippard, *The Crippled Child in New York City* (New York: Commission for the Study of Crippled Children, 1940).

7. Dorothy E. Bradbury, *Five Decades of Action for Children: A History of the Children's Bureau* (Washington, D.C.: Department of Health, Education, and Welfare, 1962).

8. For evaluations of these projects, see Karen Davis and Catherine Schoen, *Health and the War on Poverty: A Ten-Year Appraisal* (Washington, D.C.: Brookings, 1978), pp. 148–58.

9. Christa Altenstetter and James Warner Bjorkman, *Federal-State Health Policies and Impacts: The Politics of Implementation* (Washington, D.C.: University Press of America, 1978), p. 68.

10. George A. Silver, *Politics and Social Policy: Failures in Child Health Services* (New Haven: Yale University Health Policy Project, 1976), p. 28. This finding is not unique to the Title V programs. Miller and Byrne, Inc., also found in health planning, PL 93-641, that federal policy may not shift state goals. *Final Report: Evaluation of the Impact of PHS Programs on State Health Goals and Activities* (Washington, D.C.: Government Printing Office, 1977), p. 84.

11. For a complete study of Medicaid from 1965 to 1973, see Robert B. Stevens and Rosemary A. Stevens, *Welfare Medicine in America* (New York: The Free Press, 1974).

12. Mississippi was the only state to receive the maximum 83 percent reimbursement from 1966 to 1972. The states with the largest share of welfare recipients, such as California, New York, and Illinois, received the lowest matching rate, 50 percent, because of their high incomes. See, for example, *Federal Register*, 24 September 1966, pp. 12607–8; 7 September 1972, pp. 18107–8.

13. Between 1951 and 1960, medical vendor payments through public assistance rose from $48 million to $390 million. Five years later, after the enactment of Kerr-Mills, which provided greater federal support, at least to the elderly, payments had tripled to $1.3 billion. U.S. Department of Health, Education, and Welfare,

Vendor Payments for Medical Care under Public Assistance, Fiscal Years 1951–1970, NCSS Report B-7 (6 July 1971), table 7.

14. Ellen Winston, "Implications of the 1965 Amendments to the Social Security Act," *Social Work* 10 (October 1965): 12.

15. U.S. Congress, Senate, 89th Cong., 1st sess., 8 July 1965, *Congressional Record*, p. 15933.

16. PL 89-97, sec. 1902(a)(13), and 1905(a)(1) through (5).

17. James Morrison, Director, Medical Services, Connecticut State Welfare Department, interview, 26 October 1972.

18. For a lucid description of obscure bureaucratic nomenclature, see Stevens and Stevens, *Welfare Medicine in America*, pp. 61–65.

19. U.S. Department of Health, Education, and Welfare, *Medicaid Children: Who Are They?*, Social and Rehabilitation Service, 30 June 1971.

20. Advisory Commission on Intergovernmental Relations, *Intergovernmental Problems in Medicaid, A Commission Report*, September 1968, pp. 98–99.

21. PL 90-248, sec. 220(B)(1).

22. Mississippi and Alabama had maximum monthly payments to AFDC recipients of $50 to $69, while Connecticut, North Dakota, New Jersey, and New York's payment levels ranged from $230 to $256. Samuel M. Meyers and Jennie McIntyre, "Welfare Policy and Its Consequences for the Recipient Population: A Study of the AFDC Program," report submitted to the U.S. Department of Health, Education, and Welfare, Social and Rehabilitation Services, December 1969, p. 14.

23. U.S. Department of Health, Education, and Welfare, *Numbers of Recipients and Amounts of Payments Under Medicaid, 1968*, National Center for Social Statistics, report B-4 (1970), table A. (Hereafter cited as *Recipients and Payments Under Medicaid* and the year services were rendered.)

24. The number of children who received services from Medicaid during a given year is not, of course, as large as the number of children eligible to receive aid. HEW statisticians have noted considerable inconsistencies in reporting by the states. For example, California on several occasions reported more recipients than eligibles. For many years, HEW did not even attempt to find out how many eligibles there were in the nation. Even as late as 1978, all figures on needy children used by HEW and Congress were educated guesses.

25. For an excellent description of the resulting inequities of Medicaid, see Davis and Schoen, *Health and the War on Poverty*, pp. 67–83.

26. *Recipients and Payments Under Medicaid, 1969* (1972), p. 5. "Since the wealthy states also have more liberal eligibility requirements, the net result is a welfare system which rewards the rich states with far greater federal grants than those of their less affluent neighbors." Bruce Stuart, "Equity and Medicaid," *Journal of Human Resources* 7 (Spring 1972): 163.

27. Barbara S. Cooper and Mary F. McGee, "Medical Care Outlays for Three Age Groups: Young, Intermediate, and Aged," *Social Security Bulletin* 34 (May 1971): 9; Barbara S. Cooper, Nancy L. Worthington, and Paula A. Prio, "National Health Expenditures, 1929–73," *Social Security Bulletin* 37 (February 1974): 7; and HEW, *Data on the Medicaid Program: 1979 Edition (Revised)*, p. 28.

28. It has been suggested that this rise in medical care costs were due in no small part to the federal Medicaid and Medicare programs. See, for example, Karen Da-

vis, "Hospital Costs and the Medicare Program," *Social Security Bulletin* 35 (August 1973).

29. Between 1966 and 1973, the number of public assistance recipients increased from 7.4 million to 14.9 million. AFDC recipients, of whom 72 percent are children, accounted for 84 percent of this increase. U.S. Department of Health, Education, and Welfare, *Graphic Presentation of Public Assistance and Related Data*, NCSS Report A-4 (1971), p. 3, and U.S. Department of Health, Education, and Welfare, *Public Assistance Statistics*, NCSS Report A-2 (May 1973), table 1.

30. *Recipients and Payments Under Medicaid, 1970* (1972), p. 2; and U.S. Department of Health, Education, and Welfare, *Medicaid and Other Medical Care Financed from Public Assistance Funds, FY 71*, NCSS Report B-5 (November 1972), p. 2.

31. In some states an insurance company or Blue Cross acted as the fiscal agent for Medicaid. In other states the department served as its own fiscal agent.

32. Social Security Act, Section 511.

33. U.S. Congress, House, Report of Committee on Appropriations, 24 February 1943, p. 6, as cited in Nathan Sinai and Odin W. Anderson, *EMIC: A Study of Administrative Experience* (Ann Arbor: University of Michigan Press, 1948), p. 113.

34. *Ibid.*, p. 30.

35. Elizabeth A. Ingraham, "Connecticut Need for Child Hygiene Work," *Connecticut Health Bulletin* 40 (May 1926): 115.

36. Portions of the remainder of this chapter have been adapted from Anne-Marie Foltz, "The Development of Ambiguous Federal Policy: Early and Periodic Screening, Diagnosis and Treatment (EPSDT)," *Milbank Memorial Fund Quarterly/Health and Society* 53 (Winter 1975): 35–64.

37. Joseph S. Wholey, who helped direct these studies, describes the process and its pitfalls in *The Absence of Program Evaluation as an Obstacle to Effective Public Expenditure Policy: A Case Study of Child Health Care Programs* (Washington, D.C.: The Urban Institute, n.d.). The methods used are described in Arthur L. Levin, "Cost-Effectiveness in Maternal and Child Health: Implications for Program Planning and Evaluation," *New England Journal of Medicine* 278 (May 1968): 1041–47.

38. Joseph S. Wholey et al., *Program Analysis: Maternal and Child Health Care Programs* (Washington, D.C.: Department of Health, Education, and Welfare, 1966), III-22.

39. *Ibid.*, III-18.

40. At least one author of the *Program Analysis* has said that it was their intention that the program should be administered by Title V with Title XIX acting as a pass-through mechanism. Personal communication, George A. Silver, M.D., 3 June 1974.

41. U.S. Congress, Senate, 90th Cong., 1st sess., 8 February 1967, *Congressional Record*, pp. 2881–85.

42. U.S. Congress, House, Committee on Ways and Means, *Presidential Proposals for Revision in Social Security System: Hearings before the Committee on Ways and Means on H.R. 5710*, 90th Cong., 1st sess., 1–3 March 1967, p. 25. (Hereafter cited as *Hearings on H.R. 5710*.)

43. U.S. Congress, House, Committee on Ways and Means, *Section by Section Analysis and Explanation of Provisions of H.R. 5710, as Introduced on February 20, 1967*, 90th Cong., 1st sess., 1967, p. 44.

44. Sec. 1902(a)(ii) (A) and (B). (A) was the original statement; (B) was the 1967 addition.

45. *Hearings on H.R. 5710,* p. 93.

46. *Ibid.,* p. 26.

47. *Ibid.,* pp. 125–26.

48. *Ibid.,* pp. 584–85.

49. *Ibid.,* p. 2006.

50. *Ibid.,* p. 2351.

51. *Ibid.,* p. 2237.

52. *Ibid.,* p. 2242.

53. *Ibid.,* p. 2416.

54. *Ibid.,* p. 2263.

55. *Ibid.,* p. 89.

56. *Ibid.,* p. 2267.

57. *Ibid.,* p. 2229.

58. *Ibid.,* p. 1964.

59. *Ibid.,* p. 190. During 1968 (i.e., before EPSDT) the CC program served 475,000 children, while Medicaid served 5,574,000 children. The CC program had been serving over 400,000 children since 1964. No data are available on the children served by Medicaid during its first two years, 1966 and 1967. U.S. Department of Health, Education, and Welfare, *Children Who Received Physicians' Services Under the Crippled Children's Program,* MCHS Statistical Series, No. 3 (1971), table 1; and *Recipients and Payments Under Medicaid, 1968* (n.d.), table 2.

60. *Hearings on H.R. 5710,* p. 2007.

61. One major issue debated throughout the 1967 Social Security Amendments was whether the eligibility levels for medically needy should be limited to 133⅓ percent of the public assistance levels under the categorical programs. Both the states and the federal government were anxious to cut Medicaid costs by limiting the number of people who would be eligible for the medically needy category. Congress decided to apply this limitation only to the AFDC program. Consequently, the number of children eligible for EPSDT through Title XIX was curtailed by this action.

62. In fact, the MCH and CC shares, as they were allocated by the HEW Secretary, were not quite equal. The CC program received slightly more than the MCH program.

63. Social and Rehabilitation Service administrators later, when writing regulations for Title XIX, wondered whether the Title V amendment took precedence because the Title XIX amendments were "conforming." They were reassured by HEW General Counsel that juridically this had no meaning and they could proceed with regulations for Title XIX.

64. U.S. Congress, House, *Social Security Amendments of 1967: Report of the Committee on Ways and Means on H.R. 12080,* H. Rep. 544, 90th Cong., 1st sess., 1967, p. 127.

65. *Ibid.,* p. 195.

66. U.S. Congress, Senate, *Social Security Amendments of 1967: Hearings before the*

Committee on Finance, United States Senate, on H.R. 12080, 90th Cong., 1st sess., 22–24 August 1967, I, 201.

67. By 1970, this would include all states but Alaska and Arizona.

68. Proposed regulations for cooperation between Title V and Title XIX agencies had been published earlier that year but had elicited little comment from the states, possibly because the states did not know what the scope of the program would be. U.S., *Federal Register*, 4 June 1970, p. 8664.

69. *Ibid.*, 11 December 1970, pp. 18878–79.

70. Rosemary Stevens and Robert Stevens, "Medicaid: Anatomy of a Dilemma," *Law and Contemporary Problems: Health Care* 1 (Spring 1970): 365–78.

71. U.S. Congress, Senate, *Social Security Amendments of 1970: Report of the Committee on Finance, United States Senate, to Accompany H.R. 17550*, 91st Cong., 2d sess., 11 December 1970, p. 169.

72. One small midwestern state which looked more carefully at costs than others estimated that it would have fifteen to twenty children eligible for kidney dialysis at $30,000 each.

73. Two states, Virginia and Mississippi, were exceptions; they implemented the program before February 1972.

74. *Federal Register*, 11 December 1970, p. 18879. Emphasis added.

75. U.S. Department of Health, Education, and Welfare, *Medical Services State by State*, Social and Rehabilitation Service, Medical Services Administration, 801-71 (March 1971), *passim*.

76. *Federal Register*, 9 November 1971, pp. 21409–10.

77. U.S., Department of Health, Education, and Welfare, *Medicaid: Early and Periodic Screening Diagnosis and Treatment for Individuals under 21*, PRG-21, SRS, Medical Services Administration (28 June 1972).

Chapter 2

78. Gilbert Y. Steiner, *The Children's Cause* (Washington, D.C.: Brookings Institution, 1976), pp. 225–26.

79. U.S. Congress, Senate, 92d Cong., 2d sess., 30 March 1972, *Congressional Record*, p. S.5240, as cited in *ibid.*, p. 227.

80. U.S. Congress, Senate, Finance Committee, *Report to Accompany H.R. 1, Social Security Amendments of 1972*, S. Rep. 1230, 92d Cong., 2d sess., 1972, pp. 8–9. The Senate Finance Committee proposed a 2 percent penalty. This was reduced to 1 percent in the House-Senate Conference. U.S., Congress, *Conference Report to Accompany H.R. 1, Social Security Amendments of 1972*, Rep. 1605, 92d Cong., 2d sess., 1972, p. 66.

81. See, for example, U.S. Comptroller General, *Report to the Congress: Improvements Needed to Speed Implementation of Medicaid's Early and Periodic Screening, Diagnosis, and Treatment Program* (Washington, D.C.: General Accounting Office, 1975); and U.S. Congress, Senate, Senator Abraham Ribicoff, 93d Cong., 2d sess., 16 July 1974, *Congressional Record*, pp. S12574–78. Senator Ribicoff's insert in the *Record* was of a published article by John Iglehart that was highly critical of HEW.

82. U.S. Congress, House, Subcommittee on Oversight and Investigations of the Committee on Interstate and Foreign Commerce, *Report: Department of Health, Education, and Welfare's Administration of Health Programs: Shortchanging Children*, 94th Cong., 2d sess., September 1976, p. 4.

83. Children's Defense Fund, *EPSDT: Does it Spell Health Care for Children?* (Washington, D.C.: Children's Defense Fund, 1977), pp. 215–17. For an excellent analysis of the strategies and effects of these suits, see Eric Peterson, *Legal Challenges to Bureaucratic Discretion: The Influence of Lawsuits on the Implementation of EPSDT*, PB 271 040 (Springfield, Va.: National Technical Information Services, 1977).

84. "But since 1973 at my urging the Department is giving it [EPSDT] the highest priority." Department of HEW Secretary Caspar Weinberger in a speech before the National Association of Counties, Washington, D.C., 26 February 1975, as cited in *CHECK POINT—EPSDT*, no. 4 (Arlington, Va.: Human Services Institute, 1975), p. 1.

85. U.S. Department of Health, Education, and Welfare, *Understanding Medicaid: An Introduction to the Medical Services Administration* (15 May 1975), p. III.1.

86. Robert Fulton to Congressman John E. Moss, 19 October 1976. The discrepancy between Fulton and Weinberger in the citation above about the year in which EPSDT became a priority is indicative of some of the uncertainty surrounding its status. Certainly by 1975 the program was listed as a priority.

87. *Recipients and Payments Under Medicaid, 1972* (1974), p. 1; and Stevens and Stevens, *Welfare Medicine in America*, p. 243.

88. U.S. Department of Health, Education, and Welfare, *Medicaid Statistics, Fiscal Year 1976*, NCSS Report B-5 (March 1977), p. 1, and HEW, *Understanding Medicaid*, pp. IV.5–12. The counting of staff in any federal agency is always an uncertain process. One must distinguish between positions which are authorized but not necessarily filled and those which are filled. The 1972 figure given was that of positions authorized, the 1976 figure is of positions filled. Positions authorized are always greater than the number filled at any one time. However, in HEW at the time, it was not unusual to have as many as one-quarter of the authorized positions unfilled more or less permanently.

89. Keith Weikel, interview, 27 September 1977.

90. Administrator, Health Care Financing Administration, to Bruce Wolff, n.d. (c. November 1978), p. 2.

91. U.S., Department of Health, Education, and Welfare, *Medicaid FY 1978–1982: Major Program Issues*, SRS (September 1976), p. 108.

92. U.S. Congress, House, *Child Health Assessment Act: Hearings Before the Subcommittee on Health and the Environment of the Committee on Interstate and Foreign Commerce*, serial no. 95-43, 95th Cong., 1st sess., 8–9 August (*sic*) 1977, pp. 244, 266. In fact, Secretary Califano volunteered that he would take action within thirty days and report back to the Subcommittee.

93. Robert A. Derzon to the Secretary, "Operational Review of the EPSDT Program," 8 November 1977 (known as the "Rubel Report"); and Bruce S. Wolff, "HEW Program Opportunities to Expand and Enhance the Delivery of EPSDT/CHAP Services," 27 January 1978.

94. Beatrice Moore, interview, 27 September 1977.

95. Stevens and Stevens, *Welfare Medicine in America*, pp. 156–82, 260–81.

96. Estimates could be made for census income data and welfare data, but these estimates would not tell states how to identify the children.

97. U.S. Department of Health, Education, and Welfare, "Field Staff Information and Instruction Series #158: Summary of EPSDT Progress Report for Period Ending March 31, 1973," SRS, Medical Services Administration, 8 June 1973, table fol-

lowing p. 9. (Hereafter cited as "FSII Series #158.") The exact number given was 9,695,695. Some state officials have acknowledged that what they reported to the federal government was an estimate of the number of AFDC cases multiplied by the average number of children per family. For states which included medically needy and financially needy, this number was then increased by the number of children known to be eligible for other care, such as foster children. Therefore, the numbers reported would always tend to underestimate the number of children eligible in the population.

98. Anne-Marie Foltz and Donna Brown, "State Response to Federal Policy: Children, EPSDT, and the Medicaid Muddle," *Medical Care* 13 (August 1975): 637–38.

99. U.S. Congress, House, Subcommittee on Health and the Environment of the Committee on Interstate and Foreign Commerce, *Data on the Medicaid Program: Eligibility, Services, Expenditures, Fiscal Years 1966–1977* (Washington, D.C.: Government Printing Office, 1977), p. 91. This source presents data at variance with a 1977 draft document issued by the Office of Child Health, Health Care Financing Administration.

100. George D. Greenberg, "Federal Program Implementation in Selected States: A Study of the Implementation of the Partnership for Health Act and the Early and Periodic Screening, Diagnosis, and Treatment Program in Michigan, Pennsylvania, and Alabama," Report, Department of Political Science, University of Michigan, June 1979, pp. 255–65.

101. U.S. Congress, *Data on Medicaid Program, 1966–1977*, pp. 39, 89. Since Medicaid is not a direct service program, it may not be surprising that its administrative costs are so low—the range was 2 to 11 percent—compared, for example, to Public Health Service programs, which estimate administrative costs at about 20 percent of total costs. Nevertheless, Medicaid's continuing problems in monitoring fraud and abuse and administering EPSDT could be seen as a consequence of its low administrative investment.

102. Greenberg, "Federal Program Implementation in Selected States," p. 281.

103. U.S. Department of Health, Education, and Welfare, *Data on the Medicaid Program: Eligibility, Services, Expenditures Fiscal Years 1966–77*, Institute for Medicaid Management, Health Care Financing Administration, 1977, p. 102; HEW, *Data on the Medicaid Program: 1979 Edition (Revised)*, p. 104.

104. U.S. Department of Health, Education, and Welfare, "Summary of Status Reports on Early and Periodic Screening and Diagnosis and Treatment," SRS, Medical Services Administration, September 1972; and U.S. Department of Health, Education, and Welfare, "Field Staff Instruction and Information (FSII) Series, FY 74-16," SRS, Medical Services Administration, 1974, p. 1. For some reason the next quarterly report showed that only thirty-one states had a state-wide program: "FSII Series, FY 74-42."

105. U.S. Comptroller General, *Improved Administration Could Reduce the Costs of Ohio's Medicaid Program*, HRD-78-98 (Washington, D.C.: General Accounting Office, 1978), p. 139.

106. *Program Regulation Guide: EPSDT*, pp. 11–18. In one of the typical inconsistencies of federal policy these guidelines were published four months after the required implementation date of February 1972; they arrived in the states only in August of that year.

107. *Ibid.*, p. 3.

108. "FSII Series #158," p. 31. See also Bokonon Systems, Inc., *EPSDT Status: A Review of 8 States* (Washington, D.C.: Bokonon Systems, Inc., 1974), p. 81.

109. "FSII Series #158," p. 3.

110. *Program Regulation Guide: EPSDT*, p. 3.

111. "FSII Series #158," p. 3.

112. American Academy of Pediatrics, *Increased Professional Participation in State and Local EPSDT Programs* (Evanston, Ill.: American Academy of Pediatrics, 1976), p. 32.

113. "Professional Provider Participation," SRS, Medical Services Administration, unpublished data, n.d.

114. U.S. Department of Health, Education, and Welfare, " Selected Characteristics of States' EPSDT Programs," EPSDT Division, SRS, Medical Services Administration, revised April 1977 draft, p. 2.

115. AAP, *Increased Professional Participation*, p. 42.

116. *Ibid.*, p. 32. See also M. Elaine Gilliard, *Medicaid for the Young: The Early and Periodic Screening Diagnosis and Treatment Program in the South* (Atlanta: Southern Regional Council, 1976), p. 24.

117. Bokonon Systems, Inc., *EPSDT Status*, p. 70.

118. Parker Jayne to Gerry Britten, Region II EPSDT Report—Executive Summary, U.S. Department of Health, Education, and Welfare, 20 October 1976.

119. James R. Hughes, M.D., to Alfred Furoli, letter, 14 January 1976.

120. The Children's Defense Fund documented such provider problems at the sites it studied: *EPSDT*, pp. 154–60.

121. "FSII Series #158," *passim*.

122. Lindsey Bradley, Jr., "A Study of Broken Appointments for Pediatric Screening Examinations" (Master's Thesis, Trinity University, 1975), p. i; and Community Health Foundation, *A Study of Broken Appointments in the Pennsylvania EPSDT Program* (Evanston, Ill.: Community Health Foundation, 1976), p. 38.

123. HEW, "Selected Characteristics of States' EPSDT Programs," 1977 rev. draft, pp. 1, 3.

124. States using only health departments in 1975 screened 20 percent of the eligible children compared to 11 percent for states with other provider systems. Children's Defense Fund, *EPSDT*, p. 191.

125. The best study of Michigan's program is in Greenberg, "Federal Program Implementation in Selected States," pp. 154–86. Michigan also looked good because a large number of articles were published about the Michigan program by its administrators. See, for example, Avis J. Dykstra, "Michigan's Experience in the Early and Periodic Screening, Diagnosis, and Treatment Program," *American Nurses' Association Publication* NP-47 (April 1975): 43–49; Thomas R. Kirk, R. Gerald Rice, and Paul M. Allen, "EPSDT—One Quarter Million Screenings in Michigan," *American Journal of Public Health* 66 (May 1976): 482–84; Richard Currier, "Michigan Leads in Screening Medicaid-eligible Children," *Michigan Medicine* 76 (March 1977): 136–37; and Richard Currier, "EPSDT: An Experience in Preventive Health," *Urban Health* 7 (April 1978): 18–19, 56–60.

126. Foltz and Brown, "State Response to Federal Policy," p. 635.

127. U.S. Department of Health, Education, and Welfare, *Medicaid Management Reports: Annual Report, Fiscal Year 1976*, Medical Services Administration, Health Care Financing Administration, n.d., p. 24.

128. Helen Harris *et al.* vs. Thomas E. Davis *et al.*, U.S. District Court for the District of Vermont, Deposition of Joyce Morrell, 2 August 1976, pp. 19, 23.

129. James Kolb, interview, 27 September 1977.

130. The Tracer Evaluation Project found this to be the case in Michigan. Ruben Meyer *et al.*, "Tracer Evaluation of Diagnosis and Treatment of EPSDT Referrals: Final Report: Executive Summary," University of Michigan School of Public Health, December 1976, p. 13. A Texas official reported that theoretically Texas could get such data, but it came from two separate data systems, EPSDT and Medicaid, and that it would be very costly to write a new program to bring this information together. David Cook, interview, 20 February 1978.

131. Among the advocates were; Children's Defense Fund, *EPSDT*; Gilliard, *Medicaid for the Young*; and the Michigan studies cited in n. 124 above.

Among the governmental critics were: Comptroller General, *Improvements Needed to Speed Implementation of Medicaid* and *Improved Administration Could Reduce Costs of Ohio's Medicaid Program*, pp. 138–46; and House Subcommittee on Oversight and Investigations, *Shortchanging Children*.

Among the contractors were: American Management Systems, *An Evaluative Study of Early and Periodic Screening, Diagnosis, and Treatment Program in Ohio and Wisconsin* (Arlington, Va.: American Management Systems, 1974); Applied Management Sciences, *Assessment of EPSDT Practices and Costs* (Silver Springs, Md.: Applied Management Sciences, 1976); Bokonon Systems, Inc., *EPSDT Status*; Boone Young & Associates, *Revised Interim Report on Evaluation of Head Start/EPSDT Collaborative Effort* (New York: Boone Young & Assoc., 1976). The Health Services Research Institute, University of Texas, San Antonio, produced a large number of reports. Among them were: Harry W. Martin, Harold D. Dickson, *et al.*, *Impact of EPSDT—Summary. Phase II*, 1972; Fred Fielder, *Barrio Comprehensive Child Health Care Center—Final Report*, 1975; Harry W. Martin and Harold D. Dickson, *EPSDT Demonstration Projects: An Interim Evaluation, April 1974–March 1975*; Arthur E. Britt and Harold D. Dickson, *Review of Shows for Treatment: EPSDT A Nine State Survey*, 1977; Harold D. Dickson, Harry W. Martin, and Sally Davis, *Child Health in a Tri-Ethnic Rural Area—An EPSDT Demonstration in the Checkerboard Area of New Mexico*, 1978; *EPSDT Demonstration in an Urban Setting—Dallas, Texas. Final Evaluation Report*, 1978; and Harold D. Dickson, Harvey A. Evans, *et al.*, *EPSDT Diagnosis and Treatment Costs: A Five-State Analysis*, 1978.

Rigid adherence to methodology was not a hallmark of many of these studies. In 1980, the Health Policy Studies Group at Northwestern University, in an evaluation of the Health Services Research Institute work and a few other studies carried out under federal contract, judged it difficult to draw conclusions about the efficacy or effectiveness of the program because of the methods used. Janet Reis, Edward F. X. Hughes, *et al.*, *An Assessment of the Validity of the Results of HCFA's Demonstration and Evaluation Programs for the Early and Periodic Screening, Diagnosis, and Treatment Program (EPSDT): A Metaevaluation* (Evanston, Ill.: Northwestern Center for Health Policy Studies, 1980).

The few evaluations of EPSDT services which have been published in refereed professional journals include: Currier, "Michigan Leads in Screening," *Michigan Medicine*; Foltz and Brown, "State Response to Federal Policy," *Medical Care*; and Kirk, Rice, and Allen, "EPSDT in Michigan," *American Journal of Public Health*.

132. One of the confounding aspects of using such data is that in many cases the number of conditions found and referred was reported rather than the number of children who had conditions. The former may be important information, too, for it permits analysis of the conditions for which children are referred in certain states, but it confuses the reporting.

133. It was 45 percent in 1975 and 48 percent in 1978. House Subcommittee on Oversight and Investigations, *Shortchanging Children*, p. 6; and HEW, *Data on the Medicaid Program: 1979 Edition (Revised)*, pp. 52–53.

134. HEW, *Data on the Medicaid Program: 1979 Edition (Revised)*, pp. 52–53.

135. Michigan Departments of Social Services and Public Health, *EPSDT: Is Early Periodic Screening Diagnosis and Treatment Achieving Its Goal?* Report Period, January–June 1976, p. 10.

136. Minnesota Senate Health Subcommittee, *Minnesota's Progress in the EPSDT Program Development*, 21 February 1975, p. 26.

137. Children's Defense Fund, *EPSDT*, p. 139.

138. A survey in Michigan noted that the acceptance of new Medicaid patients among physicians dropped from 83.5 percent in 1973 to 68.3 percent in 1976. "Under this pressure nurses are less inclined to make referrals." Michigan Departments of Social Services and Public Health, *EPSDT*, p. 2.

139. U.S. Department of Health, Education, and Welfare, "Region I Office: Connecticut for quarters 4–5, 1976," 1976. Fiscal year 1976 had five quarters because that year the federal government transferred from a fiscal year beginning in July to one beginning in October.

140. Texas Department of Social Services, unpublished printouts.

141. *Shortchanging Children*, p. 6.

142. Britt and Dickson, *Review of Shows for Treatment: EPSDT*, p. 2. For a critique of the methods used in this study, see Children's Defense Fund, *EPSDT*, pp. 140–41.

143. *EPSDT*, p. 142, derived from data from a survey of children's records reviewed, conducted by HEW Regional Office staff. Since the Children's Defense Fund does not note how the records were chosen and since, for example, 1 percent of the records were sampled in Michigan and 30 percent in South Carolina, these results may also be methodologically suspect.

144. Wayne Stimson, *Demonstration in Follow-up: EPSDT Pierce County, Washington: Final Evaluation Report* (San Antonio: University of Texas Health Services Research Institute, 1979), p. 25.

145. HEW, *Data on the Medicaid Program, 1979 Edition (Revised)*, p. 28.

146. Davis and Schoen, *Health and the War on Poverty*, pp. 87–89.

147. For 1975: U.S. Department of Health, Education, and Welfare, National Center for Social Statistics, unpublished printouts, table 15. For 1978: Mary Tierny to Anne-Marie Foltz, personal communication, 10 April 1980. These were the costs for screening reported by the states to the federal government. Some states, in order to derive these figures, did not submit actual costs, but rather took the number of screens and multiplied them by the average amount paid by the Title XIX agency to screening providers.

148. In studying both Texas and Connecticut, I asked the states to provide the personnel data which would permit such an estimate. Connecticut, at first, could not manage a list of personnel. Texas could provide the information on personnel, but neither state could segregate the information-processing costs.

149. Applied Management Sciences, *Assessment of EPSDT Practices and Costs*, p. vii; Dickson and Evans et al., *EPSDT Diagnosis and Treatment Costs*, p. 10; Health Services Research Institute, *EPSDT Demonstration in Dallas*, p. 12.

150. Health Services Research Institute, *EPSDT Demonstration in Dallas*, p. 12. The

project received special dispensation to care for Medicaid and non-Medicaid eligible children. This made it easier to survey and reach children in the target area. It also raises a methodological question whether its results can be generalized to any other EPSDT program since such dispensation is not part of government policy.

Part II

Chapter 3

1. James L. Sundquist and David W. Davis, *Making Federalism Work* (Washington, D.C.: Brookings Institution, 1969).

2. Terry Sanford, *Storm Over the States* (New York: McGraw Hill, 1967).

3. Norman Macrae, "America's Third Century," *The Economist*, 25–31 October 1975, p. 31.

4. See, for example, Martha Derthick, *The Influence of Federal Grants* (Cambridge, Mass.: Harvard University Press, 1970).

5. One such example is the study by C. Gregory Buntz, Theodore F. Macaluso, and Jay Allen Azarow, "Federal Influence on State Health Policy," *Journal of Health Politics, Policy and Law* 3 (Spring 1978): 71–86.

6. For an excellent study of these grants, see Advisory Commission on Intergovernmental Relations, *Categorical Grants: Their Role and Design* (Washington, D.C.: Government Printing Office, 1977). See also Deil S. Wright, *Understanding Intergovernmental Relations* (North Scituate, Mass.: Duxbury Press, 1978), particularly pp. 123–79.

7. The reasons for Arizona's non-participation are complex. It has been suggested that since the majority of Arizona's poor are Indian and since the federally-funded Indian Health Service pays for *all* care for Indians on reservations, a Medicaid program might encourage poor Indians to move off the reservations and seek medical care through Medicaid. Such an event would raise Arizona's expenditures for health services, since the state would have to pick up its share of Medicaid for services which were previously paid entirely out of federal funds.

8. U.S. Department of Health, Education, and Welfare, *Handbook of Public Assistance Administration*, supplement D, appendix G, 4321, n.d.

9. Advisory Commission on Intergovernmental Relations, *Statutory and Administrative Controls Associated with Federal Grants for Public Assistance* (Washington, D.C.: Advisory Commission on Intergovernmental Relations, 1964), pp. 67–68.

10. John Holahan, William Scanlon, and Bruce Spitz, *Restructuring Federal Medicaid Controls and Incentives* (Washington, D.C.: Urban Institute, 1977), p. 74.

11. Samuel Martz, interview, 10 January 1978. Martz was a long-time participant-observer of this process, having entered government service with Social Security in the 1940s.

12. Martz, interview, 10 January 1978.

13. Galen Powers, interview, 28 September 1977.

14. Children's Defense Fund, *EPSDT: Does it Spell Health Care for Poor Children?* (Washington, D.C.: Children's Defense Fund, 1977), p. 67.

15. U.S. Comptroller General, *Improvements Needed to Speed Implementation of Medic-*

aid's Early and Periodic Screening, Diagnosis, and Treatment Program (Washington, D.C.: General Accounting Office, 1975), p. 9.

16. U.S. Congress, Senate, *Social Security Amendments of 1972: Conference Report to Accompany H.R. 1*, S. Rep. 92-1605, 92d Cong., 2d sess., 1972, p. 66.

17. PL 92-603, sec. 299F. This became Section 403g of the Social Security Act.

18. Gilbert Y. Steiner, *The Children's Cause* (Washington, D.C.: Brookings Institution, 1976), p. 230.

19. *Federal Register*, 2 August 1974, pp. 27905–7. Proposed regulations had been published six months earlier, and had elicited little comment. Only five state agencies, eight organizations, and one congressional delegation had replied. *Federal Register*, 19 December 1973, pp. 34821–22.

20. See Legal Services Organization of Indiana, "Comments on Regulations Published September 8, 1977: Child Medical Assistance Program—EPSDT Penalties," 4 November 1977, p. 1.

21. *Federal Register*, 10 August 1975, pp. 36378–80.

22. *Federal Register*, 7 September 1977, pp. 45276–82.

23. *Federal Register*, 19 May 1979, pp. 29420–27.

24. U.S. Department of Health, Education, and Welfare, "An Analysis of HCFA's December 1978 Penalty Regulations Proposal," December 1978 or January 1979, p. 1.

25. The 1974 regulations required that recipients receive screening services "within a reasonable period normally not to exceed 60 days from the date of request." *Federal Register*, 2 August 1974, p. 27905. The 1977 proposed regulations stated that screening and required treatment must be begun within 120 days. This was maintained in the regulations of 1979.

26. C. R. Weatherhogg, M.D., to John A. Svahn, Social and Rehabilitation Service Administrator, 16 September 1975, p. 1. See also part III of the present work for the controversy surrounding screening as an efficacious procedure.

27. Marion J. Woods, Director, Department of Benefit Payments, Calif., to Robert A. Derzon, Health Care Financing Administrator, 2 November 1977, p. 3.

28. Thomas M. Fawcett to Robert A. Derzon, 6 October 1977, p. 1.

29. 41 CFR, part 441.71(a)(1).

30. Keith Weikel, as quoted in John K. Iglehart, "Health Report/HEW plans to fine states for not implementing program," *National Journal*, 11 January 1975, p. 59. A children's advocate echoed the same thought: "I have problems with punishing states that do not give service to a disadvantaged population by withholding the money they use to provide other services. . . ." Gavin S. Courtney, Project Director, Citizens Committee for Children, New York City, as cited in the *New York Times*, 3 June 1975, p. 18.

31. Quoted in the *New York Times*, 8 October 1975, p. 38.

32. Children's Defense Fund, *EPSDT*, p. 68.

33. *Ibid.*

34. Galen D. Powers to James S. Dwight, Jr., "EPSDT Penalties for the First Quarter of FY 1975," 12 May 1975, p. 4.

35. James Kolb, interview, 28 September 1977.

36. Ella Grasso to James L. Martin, 18 September 1975, p. 1.

37. John T. Dempsey to Robert A. Derzon, 7 November 1977, p. 1.

38. "Memorandum," A-85 ACIR Ref. No. 75-93, 24 September 1975, p. 1.

39. *Report of Task Force on Medicaid Reform* (Washington, D.C.: National Governors' Conference, 1977), p. 17.

40. *Ibid.*, p. 3.

41. One such example is cited in Holahan, Scanlon, and Spitz, *Restructuring Medicaid*, p. 73.

42. Beatrice Moore, interview, 28 September 1977.

43. I am not here raising the issue that bureaucrats have many different things to do and that this activity was just one of many and therefore could not receive attention. That is an important constraint on any organization and does not seem unique to a federalist system.

44. During 1977 to 1978, the legislation was called the Child Health Assessment Program. By 1979, it was known as the Child Health Assurance Program. In both cases, its acronym was CHAP.

45. Beatrice Moore, interview, 1 March 1977.

46. H.R. 6706 and S. 1392, 95th Cong., 1st sess.

47. H.R. 13611, 95th Cong., 2d sess.

48. U.S., Congress, House, Committee on Interstate and Foreign Commerce, *Child Health Assurance Act of 1978*, H. Rep. 95–1481 to Accompany H.R. 13611, 95th Cong., 2d sess., 1978, p. 38.

49. Wendy Lazarus to Charles Hale Champion, 20 September 1978.

50. H.R. 4962.

Chapter 4

51. Beatrice Moore, interview, 14 March 1978; Charles Lowe, interview, 27 September 1977; George Greenberg, interview, 10 January 1978.

52. Herbert A. Simon, "On the Concept of Organizational Goals," in Amitai Etzioni, ed., *A Sociological Reader on Complex Organizations* (New York: Holt, Rinehart and Winston, 1969), p. 171.

53. Herbert A. Simon, *Administrative Behavior: A Study of Decision-Making Processes in Administrative Organizations* (New York: Free Press, 1957), pp. 199–202.

54. Anthony Downs, *Inside Bureaucracy* (Boston: Little, Brown and Co., 1967), pp. 242–43.

55. Texas agency and state libraries could make available Health Department biennial reports only since 1950, and were unable to supply Welfare Department reports for 1970, 1974, and 1977.

56. "Essentials of Public Welfare: A Statement of Principles," *Public Welfare* 11 (January 1953): 3.

57. Connecticut, *Digest of Administrative Reports to the Governor* (Hartford: Connecticut Department of Finance and Control, 1948), p. 365. (Hereafter cited as *Administrative Reports* with appropriate year.)

58. *Administrative Reports*, 1950, p. 430.

59. *Administrative Reports*, 1960, p. 264.

60. *Administrative Reports*, 1964, p. 277.

61. *Administrative Reports*, 1968, p. 306.

62. *Administrative Reports*, 1969, p. 328.

63. *Administrative Reports*, 1971, p. 336.

64. *Administrative Reports*, 1977, p. 268.

65. *Administrative Reports*, 1955, p. 166.

66. *Administrative Reports*, 1956, pp. 246–47.

67. *Ibid.*, p. 247. Improved efficiency was also a stated goal in *Administrative Reports*, 1957, p. 244.

68. *Administrative Reports*, 1969, p. 330.

69. *Administrative Reports*, 1971, p. 337.

70. *Administrative Reports*, 1976, p. 272.

71. Anne-Marie Foltz, "The Politics of Prevention: Child Health under Medicaid" (Ph.D. dissertation, Yale University, 1980), table B-4, p. 352.

72. *Administrative Reports*, 1949, p. 344.

73. *Administrative Reports*, 1948, p. 355.

74. *Administrative Reports*, 1955, p. 165.

75. *Administrative Reports*, 1960, p. 262.

76. *Administrative Reports*, 1966, p. 244.

77. *Administrative Reports*, 1967, p. 303.

78. *Administrative Reports*, 1970, p. 326.

79. *Administrative Reports*, 1971, p. 337.

80. Texas, Department of Public Welfare, *Annual Report*, 1949, p. viii. (Hereafter cited as *Welfare Report* with appropriate year.) This theme was picked up in the 1950 *Welfare Report* as well: "Democracy, we believe, cannot survive without collective concern for the individual . . . " (p. v.).

81. *Welfare Report*, 1949, p. 17.

82. *Welfare Report*, 1973, p. 3.

83. *Ibid.*, p. 5.

84. *Welfare Report*, 1972, p. 1. Emphasis in original.

85. *Welfare Report*, 1976, p. 19.

86. *Ibid.*, p. 25.

87. *Ibid.*, p. 5.

88. The worst years were immediately postwar. See the *Welfare Reports* for 1949, p. 65; 1959, p. 45; and 1960, p. 28.

89. *Welfare Reports*, 1953, p. 6; and 1962, p. 6.

90. See, for example, *Welfare Report*, 1949, p. 1; 1953, p. 6; 1971, p. 6.

91. *Welfare Report*, 1972, p. 17. The previous year ninety case workers had been transferred from social services to financial eligibility determination, which considerably limited the state's ability to give long-term social assistance.

92. Foltz, "Politics of Prevention," table B-4, p. 352.

93. *Welfare Report*, 1973, p. 21.

94. *Ibid.*, p. 17.

95. *Welfare Report*, 1975, pp. 3–4.

96. Bob Smith, interview, 24 February 1978; Marlin Johnston, interview, 23 February 1978.

97. *Welfare Report*, 1947, p. 14. Texas has 254 counties.

98. *Welfare Report*, 1954, p. 8.

99. *Welfare Report*, 1964, transmittal letter.

100. *Welfare Report*, 1966, transmittal letter.

101. *Welfare Report*, 1969, Report of the Commissioner, p. 1. This was the first change in format of the Report in many years and the first to include a Commissioner's Report reflecting on changes. The Commissioner, Burton Hackney, had been Chairman of the Board of Welfare from 1958 to 1966. After he resigned as Commissioner in 1971, this format was abandoned.

102. *Welfare Report*, 1972, p. 17.

103. *Welfare Report*, 1976, p. 9.

104. *Ibid.*, p. 13.

105. *Welfare Report*, 1973, p. 14.

106. *Welfare Report*, 1976, p. 15.

107. *Welfare Report*, 1975, pp. 3, 7. The entire report was entitled "Innovation." For example, "They showed an ability to sense needs that had not been met . . . " (p. 7).

108. Marlin Johnston, interview, 23 February 1978.

109. Stephen Press, interview, 30 March 1978.

110. "Policy Statement: The State Public Health Agency," *American Journal of Public Health* 55 (December 1965): 2011.

111. *Ibid.*

112. *Ibid.*, p. 2012.

113. *Administrative Reports*, 1947, p. 266.

114. *Administrative Reports*, 1948, p. 330.

115. Definition adopted by the House of Delegates of the American Medical Association, 2 December 1948, as cited in *Administrative Reports*, 1949, p. 305.

116. *Administrative Reports*, 1971, p. 235. Emphasis added.

117. *Ibid.*

118. *Administrative Reports*, 1959, p. 189.

119. *Administrative Reports*, 1960, p. 188. See also *Administrative Reports*, 1961, p. 185; and 1969, p. 243.

120. *Administrative Reports*, 1967, p. 235.

121. R. M. Gibson and C. R. Fisher, "National Health Expenditures, Fiscal Year 1977," *Social Security Bulletin* 4 (July 1976): 3–20, as cited in U.S., Department of Health, Education, and Welfare, *Health: United States, 1978*, Pub. No. 78-1232 (December 1978), pp. 380, 383.

122. Foltz, "Politics of Prevention," table B-4, p. 352.

123. *Administrative Reports*, 1967, pp. 216–17.

124. *Administrative Reports*, 1950, p. 396.

125. *Administrative Reports*, 1951, p. 292.

126. *Administrative Reports*, 1961, p. 192.

127. *Administrative Reports*, 1968, p. 226.

128. *Ibid.*

129. *Administrative Reports*, 1977, p. 198.

130. *Ibid.*

131. "Staff also participated in activities related to the Department of Social Services Panel on Title XIX, and to early and periodic screening, diagnosis and treatment of children." *Administrative Reports*, 1976, p. 204. See also *Administrative Reports*, 1974, p. 232.

132. *Administrative Reports*, 1974, p. 230. The regulations were actually adopted by the Public Health Council, which was legally responsible for department policy. In fact, most of the work was done by the department itself. By the end of the 1970s the Public Health Council itself had been eliminated as an anachronism, with the Commissioner of Health receiving the regulatory power held by the council.

133. Texas Department of Health, *Biennial Report*, 1950–52, p. 8. (Hereafter cited as *Biennial Report* with appropriate years.) See also *Biennial Report*, 1954–56, p. 8: that the State Health Department "is the official governmental agency charged with the responsibility of protecting and promoting the health of all the people of this state."

134. *Biennial Report*, 1950–52, p. 73.

135. *Biennial Report*, 1952–54, p. 16. This goal was reiterated in the *Biennial Report*, 1960–62, p. 75.

136. *Biennial Report*, 1952–54, p. 8.

137. Hal L. Harle, interview, 22 February 1978; Jean Shoemaker, interview, 24 February 1978; Ray Kruger, interview, 24 February 1978.

138. *Biennial Report*, 1950–52, p. 25.

139. *Biennial Report*, 1958–60, p. 49.

140. *Biennial Report*, 1968–70, p. 84.

141. *Biennial Report*, 1975–77, p. 13. The report for 1970–72 states: "Responsibilities of the regional operations include: (a) supporting all health programs that are operating within the region; (b) provide comprehensive public health services to all people within the region; (c) provide assistance to organized health units within the region; (d) provide health planning assistance to all governmental and private agencies; (e) to develop, coordinate, and implement active education programs in all areas." (*Biennial Report*, 1970–72, p. 81.) Descriptions of what the regions did were given in subsequent reports.

142. *Biennial Report*, 1950–52, p. 8; and 1954–56, p. 9.

143. *Biennial Report*, 1952–54, p. 27.

144. *Ibid.*, p. 73.

145. *Biennial Report*, 1956–58, pp. 23–24.

146. *Biennial Report*, 1968–70, p. 15; and 1970–72, p. 15.

147. *Biennial Report*, 1954–56, p. 8.

148. *Biennial Report*, 1956–58, p. 8.

149. *Ibid.*

150. Foltz, "Politics of Prevention," table B-4, p. 352.

151. *Biennial Report*, 1952–54, p. 24.

152. "The primary functions of the Venereal Disease Division are to act in an advisory and supervisory capacity to local communities. . . ." *Ibid.*, p. 73.

153. *Biennial Report*, 1968–70, p. 15. A similar statement appeared in the following *Biennial Report*, 1970–72, p. 15.

154. *Biennial Report*, 1956–58, p. 49.

155. For example, the establishment of cancer clinics to train physicians (*Biennial Report*, 1950–52, p. 22) and nurse continuing education programs in "Basic Public Health Nursing" (*Biennial Report*, 1975–77, p. 82).

156. *Biennial Report*, 1958–60, p. 16.

157. *Biennial Report*, 1960–62, p. 101; and 1966–68, p. 17.

158. *Biennial Report*, 1950–52, p. 15; and 1960–62, p. 117. By 1968–70, migrants were added to the group receiving direct services: *Biennial Report*, p. 116.

159. *Biennial Report*, 1975–77, p. 56.

160. *Biennial Report*, 1966–68, p. 31.

Chapter 5

161. Anne-Marie Foltz and Donna Brown, "State Response to Federal Policy: Children, EPSDT, and the Medicaid Muddle," *Medical Care* 13 (August 1975): 630–42.

162. Beatrice Moore, interview, 27 September 1977; and Chapin Wilson, interview, 28 September 1977.

163. U.S. Congress, Senate, *Social Security Amendments of 1970: Report of the Committee on Finance to Accompany H.R. 17550*, S. Rep. 91-1431, 91st Cong., 2d sess., 11 December 1970, p. 105.

164. This idea first appeared in *Task Force on Medicaid and Related Programs, Report* (Washington, D.C.: Government Printing Office, 1970), pp. 68–69. This was also known as the *McNerney Report*, after the Task Force's Chairman.

165. PL 92-603, sec. 235.

166. HEW, *Data on the Medicaid Program, 1979 Edition (Revised)*, p. 104.

167. Henrietta Duvall, interview, 9 September 1977. The General Accounting Office was highly critical of these subsystems and their efficacy. U.S. Comptroller General, *Attainable Benefits of the Medicaid Management Information System Are Not Being Realized*, HRD 78-151 (Washington, D.C.: General Accounting Office, 1978), pp. 31–44.

168. Wesley Amend, interview, 27 September 1977.

169. *Recipients and Payments under Medicaid*, 1970, table 1.

170. American Medical Association, *Distribution of Physicians, Hospitals and Hospital Beds in the U.S., 1972*, I (Chicago: American Medical Association, 1972).

171. Anne-Marie Foltz, "The Impact of Federal Child Health Policy Under EPSDT: The Case of Connecticut," Yale Health Policy Project, Report No. 3, Yale University Department of Epidemiology and Public Health, New Haven, 1974, p. 21.

172. Foltz and Brown, "State Response to Federal Policy," pp. 634–35.

173. Foltz, "Impact of Policy Under EPSDT," appendix tables 4A, 4B.

174. Foltz and Brown, "State Response to Federal Policy," p. 635.

175. In 1976, only 63 percent of physicians in the state were actually receiving payments for seeing Medicaid patients, and of these 42 percent were paid less than $500 during the year, a sign they did not have a very active Medicaid practice.

Patricia Day, Chief, Research and Statistics of Social Services, to Stephen Press, Director, Health Services, Department of Social Services, "Medicaid Billings," 21 September 1977.

176. The Welfare Department would at irregular intervals issue updated lists of EPSDT providers. The term "EPSDT provider" is a misnomer since it refers to a provider only of screening, despite the acronym, which would indicate the provider did more. In fact, any physician who had a Medicaid provider number could diagnose and treat an eligible child and be paid by Medicaid. He could also include most of the screening tests, but if he billed under his Medicaid number, no one would ever know that the child had been screened. On the other hand, the local public nursing agencies could only screen.

177. Stephen Locke, interview, 12 December 1977; Harold McIntosh, interview, 12 December 1977; Stephen Press, interview, 30 March 1978.

178. Stephen W. Locke to Joan R. Kemler, "Draft of Revised Implementation Plan for MMIS," Department of Social Services, 9 March 1978.

179. Brian McCarthy, interview, 3 May 1978. The FS 2082s were the basic HEW form on which the federal agency based all its reporting on services. Despite my repeated requests to receive more recent and presumably more reliable data, the department was unable to provide them during 1978. Even data from the monthly NCSS 120 forms on EPSDT screening for 1976 and 1977 contained inconsistencies and internal errors. These reports were also at variance with what Washington reported for the state during the same period.

180. Estelle Siker, interview, 1 February 1978.

181. Harold McIntosh, interview, 12 December 1977; and Community Health Foundation, "Basic Issues in the Development of the Connecticut EPSDT Program," Evanston, Ill., 11 March 1977, p. 5. In 1973–1974, staff in the medical payments office as a whole was cut by 31 percent, so although the assignment of 1.1 persons does not seem like much, at least it was an acknowledgement of a need to staff the program. Foltz, "Impact of Policy Under EPSDT," p. 19.

182. Harold McIntosh, "Deposition," Economic Rights Organization (ERO) et al. vs. Edward W. Maher, Commissioner of Social Services et al., U.S. Dist. Ct., Dist. of Conn., Civil Action No. N-78-483, 29 December 1978, pp. 5–6.

183. Morris A. Wessel, interview, Fall 1974.

184. "Development of the Connecticut EPSDT Program," p. 7.

185. Stephen Press, "Deposition," ERO et al. vs. Maher et al., 2 January 1979, p. 4.

186. The CETA program, as its name implies, was designed to provide training for the unemployed and then place them in regular permanent jobs; the funds, under federal law, could not be used for the same positions for more than a year.

187. "Deposition," ERO et al. vs. Maher et al., 2 January 1979, p. 25. The legislator in question, Joan Kemler, said, "All these workers do is make about one phone call a day. I can't justify institutionalizing new department positions in a program like that." Cited in the Hartford Courant, 30 April 1978, p. 27. She had also cut department staff investigating fraud and abuse, saying that the department did not need the investigators (ibid.).

188. Alfred G. Fuoroli to Edward W. Maher, 27 November 1978.

189. Connecticut Department of Social Services, "All Eligible Persons for the Period from July 1, 1977 thru June 30, 1978."

190. Stephen Press, interview, 30 March 1978.

191. HEW, *Data on the Medicaid Program, 1979 Edition (Revised)*, table 26.

192. Foltz and Brown, "State Response to Federal Policy," p. 635.

193. HEW, *Recipients and Payments Under Medicaid, 1970*, table 1.

194. Texas Department of Health Resources, "Counties With No or Fewer than Recommended Physicians Within Designated Population Ranges," March 1977.

195. Ray Kruger, interview, 25 February 1978.

196. Dental care was a mandated part of the EPSDT program. Before EPSDT, Texas, unlike Connecticut, had not provided dental care to children under its optional services. Therefore, the state set up a separate dental program for children under twenty-one as part of the EPSDT operation. This was part of the contract to the Health Department and ended up taking a greater share of EPSDT funds than did the screening. For example, in 1977, the Health Department spent $11 million for dental care and $3 million for screening out of its $16 million EPSDT contract. Texas, Department of Health Resources, "Report on Expenditures and Encumbrances FY 1977 For the Period 9-1-76 through 8-1-77; EPSDT Contract—TDH and DHR As of 12-31-77."

197. Marlin Johnston, interview, 23 February 1978.

198. S. J. Lerro, M.D., testimony in Texas Department of Public Welfare, Blue Ribbon Task Force for the Evaluation of Medicaid in Texas, Special Medical Services Subcommittee, *Expert Legislative and Staff Testimony*, 15 February 1977, p. 11-185.

199. For a description of how the program worked in its early months, see Ann Maravilla, "The Early and Periodic Screening, Diagnosis, and Treatment Program (EPSDT): Lessons from a 10-month Experience in North Texas," *Clinical Pediatrics* 16 (February 1977): 173–78.

200. Charlene Chunk Cavett, interview, 22 February 1978.

201. Hal L. Harle, interview, 22 February 1978; Dorothy Casey, interview, 23 February 1978.

202. "Summary of Average Cost per Screen for Year Ending 8/31/78 as of 12/31/77," p. 1.

203. Lerro, testimony before the Special Medical Services Subcommittee, p. 11-209.

204. Texas Department of Public Welfare, Task Force for the Evaluation of Medicaid in Texas, *Final Report: Recommendations and Issues* (Austin: Department of Public Welfare, 1977), p. 25.

205. Victor Kugajevsky and Allan Lazar, "Controlling Eligibility Errors in the Medicaid Program," *Journal for Medicaid Management* 1 (Summer 1977): 10–11.

206. Robert Tyndall, "An Overview of the Texas Recipient Health Care Education Program," in Pacific Consultants, eds., *Patient and Provider Profiling (S/UR): Conference Summary* (Washington, D.C.: Department of Health, Education, and Welfare, Institute for Medicaid Management, 1977), pp. 238–43.

207. U.S. Department of Health, Education, and Welfare, "Federal Dollars Paid to the States (as of 12/31/77) for MMIS Development and Operation," table 1.

208. David Cooke, personal communication, March 1978. Cooke noted that these estimates may have been low: "Due to the structure of our accounting system, it is difficult to break out MMIS expenditures."

209. Bob Smith, interview, 24 February 1978.

210. The exact number varied from year to year and not all positions allocated were filled, so that some regions were better served than others. For example, a

1976 HEW Regional Office report noted a problem in the San Antonio area: Mike Notzon to Ross Clinchy, "Trip Report—April 2, 1976—EPSDT, Family Planning, Transportation," 26 April 1976, p. 3. With about 450 workers and about 333,000 children eligible, each worker had responsibility for 740 children.

211. Bob Smith, interview, 24 February 1978; Charlene Chunk Cavett, interview, 22 February 1978.

212. Jean Shoemaker, interview, 24 February 1978.

213. Armondo Figueroa, questioning Dr. Lerro, testimony before the Special Medical Services Subcommittee, p. 11-202.

214. Bob Smith, interview, 21 February 1978.

215. William Pierce, interview, 24 February 1978.

216. See, for example, the testimony of Dr. John Smith, president-elect of the Texas Medical Association, Blue Ribbon Task Force for the Evaluation of Medicaid, Physicians' Subcommittee, *Provider Testimony*, 31 January 1977, pp. 24–30.

217. Charlene Chunk Cavett, interview, 22 February 1978.

218. Ray Kruger, interview, 25 February 1978. The department had to count these manually because the computer system was still not capable of generating these data. Moreover, the data had to come either from the physician or the case worker referral form. If the physician treated, returned no referral form, and billed on his Medicaid number, neither the Health nor Welfare Department would know that the child had received care because the Medicaid billing system was separate from the EPSDT data system.

219. Bob Smith, interview, 21 February 1978. The screening cost itself was an additional $18 to $24.

220. Charlene Chunk Cavett, interview, 22 February 1978.

221. Hal L. Harle, interview, 22 February 1978. On the other hand, the nurses in the EPSDT clinics could simply hand the mothers a bottle of Kwell and explain its use.

222. Marlin Johnston, interview, 23 February 1978. Others in their interviews who commented on both the power of the Texas Medical Association and on its unwillingness to let public agencies treat people were Jean Shoemaker, Ray Kruger, Arthur Britt, David Warner, and Hal L. Harle.

Part III

Chapter 6

1. Charles Lewis, tongue in cheek, combined definitions from three sources—the World Health Organization, Julius Richmond, and Helen Wallace—to come up with a definition of comprehensive care as: "*Coordinated, Continuing, Accessible, Optimal, Personal, Medical* (preventive, curative, rehabilitative), *Social, Dental, Emotional, Educational, Vocational, Nutritional, Recreational* Services rendered by *Team* focused on Family as unit." (Emphases in original.) "Does Comprehensive Care Make a Difference?", *American Journal of Diseases of Children* 122 (December 1971): 469. Evaluators of health programs have tended to use the term to mean a program including preventive and curative services given at one site. See, for example, Joel J. Alpert, Margaret Heagerty, *et al.*, "Effective Use of Comprehensive Pediatric Care," *American Journal of Diseases of Children* 116 (November 1968): 529–33; Leon Gordis and Milton Markowitz, "Evaluation of the Effectiveness of Com-

prehensive and Continuous Pediatric Care," *Pediatrics* 48 (November 1971): 766–76; and Barbara M. Korsch, Vida F. Negrete, *et al.*, "How Comprehensive are Well Child Visits?", *American Journal of Diseases of Children* 122 (December 1971): 483–88.

2. "The services, not the specialty of the provider, form the basis of this definition of primary care." Institute of Medicine, *Interim Report of a Study: Primary Care in Medicine: A Definition* (Washington, D.C.: National Academy of Sciences, 1977), p. 1.

3. U.S. Congress, House, Subcommittee on Health and the Environment of the Committee on Interstate and Foreign Commerce, *A Discursive Dictionary of Health Care*, 94th Cong., 2d sess., February 1976, p. 127.

4. M. F. Hansen and Carolyn Aradine, "The Changing Face of Primary Pediatrics: Review and Commentary," *Pediatric Clinics of North America* 21 (February 1974): 246. The training of physicians for primary care has been particularly emphasized, as in the Institute of Medicine, *Interim Report*, and David E. Rogers, "The Challenge of Primary Care," *Daedalus: Doing Better and Feeling Worse: Health in the United States* 106 (Winter 1977): 82. Archie S. Golden, *An Inventory for Primary Health Care Practice* (Cambridge, Mass.: Ballinger, 1976), lays out the tasks which must be carried out in primary care.

5. For example, George Rosen states, "Preventive medicine has never been a popular subject among medical students or medical practitioners," in *Preventive Medicine in the United States 1900–1975* (New York: Science History Publications, 1975), p. 52. For the formation of preventive medicine as a medical specialty, see Rosemary Stevens, *American Medicine and the Public Interest* (New Haven: Yale University Press, 1971), pp. 330–31.

6. See Commission on Chronic Illness, *Chronic Illness in the United States* I (Cambridge, Mass.: Harvard University Press, 1957), p. 45; R. M. Thorner and Q. R. Remein, *Principles and Procedures in the Evaluation of Screening for Disease*, Monograph #67 (Washington, D.C.: Public Health Service, 1961), pp. 2–12; Thomas McKeown, "Validation of Screening Procedures," in McKeown, ed., *Screening in Medical Care: Reviewing the Evidence*, Nuffield Provincial Hospitals Trust (London: Oxford University Press, 1968), pp. 1–13; J. M. G. Wilson and G. Jungner, *Principles and Practices of Screening for Disease*, Public Health Paper #34 (Geneva: World Health Organization, 1968), pp. 11–39; A. L. Cochrane and W. W. Holland, "Validation of Screening Procedures," *British Medical Bulletin* 27 (1971): 3–8; L. Whitby, "Screening Definitions and Criteria," *Lancet* 2 (5 October 1974): 819–21. For a study of application of these criteria to a screening program, see Anne-Marie Foltz and Jennifer L. Kelsey, "The Annual Pap Test: A Dubious Policy Success," *Milbank Memorial Fund Quarterly/Health and Society* 56 (Fall 1978): 426–62.

7. W. W. Holland, "Screening: Taking Stock," *Lancet* 2 (December 1974): 1494–96.

8. Rene Dubos devotes a chapter to this theme and John Gordon Freymann refers to it as the "great schism." Rene Dubos, *Mirage of Health* (New York: Harper and Row, 1959), pp. 129–69; John Gordon Freymann, "Medicine's Great Schism: Prevention vs. Cure: An Historical Interpretation," *Medical Care* 13 (July 1975): 525–36.

9. Innovation and progress are not necessarily synonymous, although Alexis de Tocqueville noted in the early nineteenth century that Americans tended to equate them. *Democracy in America* I (New York: Vintage Books, 1955), p. 443.

10. So strong had this expectation become that by 1978 the press had taken to reminding the public that everything is not curable; everyone must take risks and at some time die. See, for example, Michael S. Kramer, "My Turn: The Risks of Health," *Newsweek*, 6 February 1978, p. 11.

11. J. M. G. Wilson, "The Worth of Detecting Occult Disease," in C. L. E. H. Sharp and Harry Keen, eds., *Presymptomatic Detection and Early Diagnosis: A Critical Appraisal* (London: Pittman and Sons, 1968), p. 144.

12. Julian Tudor Hart cites one exception: "The greatest number of lives saved by any screening procedure must surely have been during the 1914–1918 war, when almost any loud systolic murmer was diagnosed as valvular disease of the heart, and disqualified a man for the trenches." "Screening in Primary Care," in Cyril J. R. Hart, ed., *Screening in General Practice* (Edinburgh: Churchill Livingstone, 1975), p. 18. Hart fails to note that someone else had to take the lucky "diseased" man's place in the trenches.

13. Iago Galdston noted the importance of the introduction of the periodic exam for the physician which "promises to deeply affect the relations of patient and physician, restoring the general practitioner to his former position as family friend, confidant, and advisor." He added that insurance companies with their objectives of maintaining the physical health and prolonging the lives of their policyholders could form a powerful combination for the investigation of health problems. "The Genealogy of the Health Examination," *The Health Examiner* 1 (February 1932): 7, 10.

14. Rosen, *Preventive Medicine*, p. 59.

15. *Ibid.*, p. 60.

16. Committee on the Cost of Medical Care, *Medical Care for the American People: The Final Report* (Chicago: University of Chicago Press, 1932; reprint ed., Washington, D.C.: U.S. Health Services and Mental Health Administration, Community Health Service, 1970), p. 42.

17. S. Charles Franco, "The Early Detection of Disease by Periodic Examination," *Industrial Medicine and Surgery* 25 (June 1956): 251–57; Kendall A. Elsom, Stanley Spoont, and H. Phelps Potter, "An Appraisal of the Periodic Health Examination," *Industrial Medicine and Surgery* 25 (August 1956): 367–71.

18. Charles E. Thompson, Earl A. Zaus, and Philip R. Keller, "Some Observations on Periodic Health Examinations," *Journal of Occupational Medicine* 3 (April 1961): 215–17. On p. 217 the authors cite three studies in addition to the Franco one noted above.

19. *Ibid.*, p. 217.

20. Some of these studies which showed favorable mortality rates among executives compared to the general public, suffered from methodological weaknesses in their choice of comparison groups. See, for example, Robert M. Thorner and E. L. Crumpacker, "Mortality and Periodic Examinations of Executives," *Archives of Environmental Health* 3 (November 1961): 523–25.

21. This periodic assessment was known as the multiphasic health checkup, which meant that a battery of multiple screening tests was administered by technicians who then relayed the results to physicians for final evaluation. Multiphasic screening programs had a brief vogue, but did not become regular practice in most areas of the country. They were established on the assumption that they would be more cost-effective than assessments by physicians alone.

22. Morris F. Collen, "A Cast Study of Multiphasic Health Testing," in National Academy of Sciences, *Medical Technology and the Health Care System: A Study of Equipment-Embodied Technology.* Report by the Committee on Technology and Health Care, Assembly of Engineering, National Research Council and Institute of Medicine (Washington, D.C.: National Academy of Sciences, 1978), p. 150.

23. David L. Sackett and W. W. Holland, "Controversy in the Detection of Disease," *Lancet* 2 (23 August 1975): 358.

24. Stanley S. Schor *et al.*, "An Evaluation of the Periodic Health Examination: The findings in 350 examinees who died," *Annals of Internal Medicine* 61 (November 1964): 999–1005.

25. Jack R. Harnes, "Second and Subsequent Periodic Examinations," *New York State Journal of Medicine* 76 (June 1976): 896.

26. Morris Collen, "Periodic Health Examination: Why? What? When? How?", *Primary Care* 3 (1976): 201. See also his earlier "Automated Multiphasic Screening" in Sharp and Keen, eds., *Detection and Early Diagnosis*, pp. 25–66. Other believers were those who promoted, for example, the annual Pap test for women. See H. K. Fidler, D. A. Boyes, and A. J. Worth, "Screening for Malignant Disease by Means of Exfoliative Cytology," in Sharp and Keen, eds., *Detection and Early Diagnosis*, pp. 295–333.

  Among the early skeptics were A. L. Cochrane and P. C. Elwood, "Medical Scientists look at Screening," in Sharp and Keen, eds., *Detection and Early Diagnosis*, pp. 359–66. Later skeptics included: Thomas L. DelBlanco, "The Periodic Health Examination for the Adult: Waste or Wisdom," *Primary Care* 3 (June 1976): 205–14; Walter O. Spitzer and Bruce P. Brown, "Unanswered Questions about the Periodic Health Examination," *Annals of Internal Medicine* 83 (1975): 257–63; and Lewis Thomas, "On the Science and Technology of Medicine," *Daedalus* 106 (Winter 1977): 35–46.

27. Richard Spark, "The Case against Regular Physicals," 25 July 1976, pp. 10–11, 38–41.

28. Collen, "Periodic Health Examinations," p. 199.

29. These arguments, presented since the early 1900s, were echoed in a report in 1977: U.S. Department of Health, Education, and Welfare, Office of Child Health Affairs, *A Proposal for New Federal Leadership in Child and Maternal Health Care in the United States*, 23 February 1977, pp. 2–6. This document also added a fourth reason, "equal opportunity."

30. See, for example, T. M. Rotch, *Pediatrics*, 3rd ed. (Philadelphia: J. P. Lippincott Co., 1903), a pediatric textbook that stressed, "in no period of life is prophylaxis of disease so important and the results so variant as in infancy and early childhood," as cited in Hugh C. Thompson, "Preventive Services for Children," *Pediatric Clinics of North America* 16 (1969): 947.

31. Helen M. Dart, *Maternity and Child Care in Selected Rural Areas of Mississippi*, Pub. 88 (Washington, D.C.: U.S. Children's Bureau, 1921), as cited in Robert H. Bremner, ed., *Children and Youth in America: A Documentary History*, 3 vols. (Cambridge, Mass.: Harvard University Press, 1970–1974), 2:973; and J. H. Mason Knox, "Morbidity and Mortality in the Negro Infant," *Transactions of the American Pediatric Society* 36 (1924), as cited in Bremner, ed., *Children and Youth*, 2:975.

32. See, for example, Martha M. Eliot, "A Demonstration of the Community Control of Rickets," *Child Health Bulletin* 2 (1926): 38–44, as cited in Bremner, ed., *Children and Youth*, 2:1074–76.

33. Whether this was just a strategy to promote a health program for crippled children as a piece of political opportunism is not entirely clear. The proponents of health services for children in 1935 believed that if a general program failed, at least one directed toward crippled children would meet the approval and interest of a president who was himself crippled. The result was the crippled children's

provisions of the Social Security Act. See Edwin E. Witte, *The Development of the Social Security Act* (Madison: University of Wisconsin Press, 1963), p. 171.

34. *Child Health Services and Pediatric Education: Report of the Committee for the Study of Child Health Services* (New York: Commonwealth Fund, 1949), p. 20.

35. Joseph Wholey *et al.*, *Program Analysis: Maternal and Child Health Care Programs* (Washington, D.C.: U.S. Department of Health, Education, and Welfare, 1966), p. II.4.

36. *Ibid.*, pp. II.7–11.

37. American Academy of Pediatrics, *Lengthening Shadows: A Report of the Council on Pediatric Practice* (Evanston, Ill.: American Academy of Pediatrics, 1970), pp. 14–15.

38. See, for example, National Council of Organizations for Children and Youth, *America's Children, 1976* (Washington, D.C.: National Council of Organizations for Children and Youth, 1976), pp. 32, 36, 40–44.

39. *Pediatrics* 20 (1908): 580–81, as cited in Bremner, ed., *Children and Youth*, 2:1058–59.

40. Bremner, ed., *Children and Youth*, 3:113. Among non-college-bound youth eighteen years old, 15 percent were rejected by the Selective Service Board for handicapping conditions of which 62 percent were preventable. Wholey *et al.*, *Program Analysis*, p. II.8 and table 2.7.

41. A. L. Cochrane refers to effectiveness as measuring the "effect of a particular medical action in altering the natural history of a particular disease for the better." *Effectiveness and Efficiency* (London: Oxford University Press for Nuffield Provincial Hospitals Trust, 1972), p. 2.

42. Rosen, *Preventive Medicine*, pp. 5–6. See also Martha M. Eliot, "Emergency Food Relief and Child Health," 1931, cited in Bremner, ed., *Children and Youth*, 2:1083–88.

43. Rosen, *Preventive Medicine*, p. 49.

44. New York City extended this instruction to young girls, as well, in its "Little Mothers' Leagues." U.S. Department of Health, Education, and Welfare, *Child Health in America*, Pub. (HSA) 5015 (Washington, D.C.: Government Printing Office, 1976), p. 32.

45. White House Conference on Child Health and Protection, 1930, *Health Protection for the Preschool Child*, cited in Bremner, ed., *Children and Youth*, 2:1082.

46. Rosen, *Preventive Medicine*, p. 44. Whether this precipitous decline can be attributed solely to the antitoxin is debatable. Improved sanitation, housing, and nutrition were certainly factors as well.

47. This assumption is implicit, for example, in the use of hospitalization for rheumatic fever as an outcome variable in the evaulation of comprehensive care programs in Baltimore. See Leon Gordis, "Effectiveness of Comprehensive Care Programs in Preventing Rheumatic Fever," *New England Journal of Medicine* 289 (16 August 1973): 372–73.

48. Tay-Sachs and other types of genetic screening have generated some controversy. On Tay-Sachs, see *New England Journal of Medicine* 291:1166–70; 292:371 and 758; and 295:113. The ethical issue here is whether knowledge of being a carrier of Tay-Sachs is an advantage and whether people want to know whether or not they are carriers. Other genetic screening programs, such as screening for sickle cell trait, have also aroused controversy since those detected with the trait may be la-

beled erroneously as handicapped. See Marc Lappe *et al.*, "Ethical and Social Is-sues in Screening for Genetic Disease," *New England Journal of Medicine* 286 (25 May 1972): 1129–32; and Amitai Etzioni, *Genetic Fix* (New York: Harper and Row, 1973).

49. Holger Hansen, "Prevention of Mental Retardation Due to PKU: Selected As-pects of Program Validity," *Preventive Medicine* 4(1975): 310–21.

50. John B. Blake, *Origins of Maternal and Child Health Programs* (New Haven: Yale School of Medicine, 1953), pp. 28–30.

51. Hugh C. Thompson and Joseph B. Seagle, *The Management of Pediatric Practice: A Philosophy and Guide* (Springfield, Ill.: Charles C. Thomas, 1961), p. 128.

52. American Academy of Pediatrics, *Child Health Services* pp. 50–51. By contrast, general practitioners who were physicians for the less wealthy, and in rural areas, saw well children for only 30 percent of visits.

53. Alfred Yankauer *et al.*, "Pediatric Practice in the United States," *Pediatrics* 45 supplement (March 1970): 524. Morris Green and Julius Richmond stated that 60 to 80 percent of a pediatrician's time was spent in preventive care, but gave no source for that statement. *Pediatric Diagnosis*, 2d ed. (Philadelphia: W. B. Saunders, 1962), p. 439.

54. Arlen L. Rosenbloom and James P. Ongley, "Who Provides What Services to Children in Private Medical Practice?", *American Journal of Diseases of Children* 127 (March 1974): 357–61. The authors also noted that one-half of the pediatricians' well-child visits were for children under two years old, suggesting "maldistributed attention" (p. 360).

55. Alfred Yankauer and Ruth Lawrence, "A Study of Periodic School Medical Ex-aminations: II. The Annual Increment of New Defects," *American Journal of Public Health* 46 (December 1956): 1559.

56. F. P. Anderson, "Evaluation of the Routine Physical Examination of Infants in the First Year of Life," *Pediatrics* 45 (1970): 950–60.

57. Robert A. Hoekelman, "What Constitutes Adequate Well-baby Care?", *Pediat-rics* 55 (March 1975): 313–26. See also letters generated by this article in *Pediatrics* 58 (October 1976): 627–29 and (November 1976): 772.

58. The extensive and careful Rochester ambulatory care controlled experiment showed that the program of comprehensive care (preventive and curative) to low-income children resulted in fewer illness visits, increased health supervision visits, lower hospitalization rates, and increased satisfaction. Morbidity was, however, unaffected. Joel J. Alpert *et al.*, "Effective Use of Comprehensive Pediatric Care," *American Journal of Diseases of Children* 116 (November 1968): 529–33; and Joel J. Al-pert *et al.*, "Delivery of Health Care for Children: Report of an Experiment," *Pediat-rics* 57 (June 1976): 917–30.

Similar controlled experiments carried out in Baltimore on infants of teenage mothers indicated no differences in morbidity between children receiving continu-ous care and episodic illness-related care. However, the short duration of the study (fifteen months) may have influenced the findings. Gordis and Markowitz, "Evaluation of the Effectiveness of Pediatric Care," pp. 766–76.

59. New York Academy of Medicine *Bulletin* 51 (January 1975).

60. See, for example, Robert H. Brook, "Quality of Care Assessment: Policy Rele-vant Issues," *Policy Sciences* 5 (1974): 317–41; Allyson Davies Avery *et al.*, *Quality of Medical Care Assessment Using Outcome Measures: Eight Disease-Specific Applications* (Santa Monica, Calif.: Rand, 1976); and Hyman K. Schonfeld, Jean F. Heston, and Isadore S. Falk, *Standards for Good Medical Care Based on the Opinions of Clinicians*

Associated with the Yale-New Haven Medical Center with Respect to 242 Diseases, PB-240-385 (Springfield, Va.: National Technical Information Service, 1975).

61. Epidemiologists have pointed out that the distributions of findings on any test tend to follow a bell-shaped curve. Where one moves from the normal to abnormal is a matter of definition, not necessarily a question of health. Thus, the existence of diseases such as diabetes or glaucoma must be reviewed in relative terms. Moreover, it is not a medically logical conclusion that someone whose test readings falls outside two standard deviations from the mean is actually suffering from a disease that needs treatment. See Thorner and Remein, *Principles and Procedures*; Wilson and Jungner, *Principles and Practices*; Sackett and Holland, "Controversy in the Detection of Disease"; and A. L. Cochrane, "The History of the Measurement of Ill Health," *International Journal of Epidemiology* 1 (1972): 89–92.

62. David Kessner, Carolyn Kalk Show, and James Singer, *Assessment of Medical Care for Children* (Washington, D.C.: Institute of Medicine, National Academy of Sciences, 1974), pp. 27, 76–77. The authors found that few of the children with low hematocrits were treated, but dismissed the idea that the health providers in the study did not accept their criteria for anemia because the criteria had been established with the assistance of clinicians and researchers (p. 77). For an excellent review of the literature on iron-deficiency anemia, see Barbara Starfield, "Iron-Deficiency Anemia," Harvard Child Health Project, vol. 2: *Children's Medical Care Needs and Treatment* (Cambridge, Mass.: Ballinger, 1977), pp. 77–120.

63. Grace Abbot, introduction to "Organizing for Administration of Child Welfare Services," in *The Child and the State*, vol. 2 (Chicago: University of Chicago Press, 1938); reprinted in Bremner, ed., *Children and Youth*, 2:755.

64. Gilbert Y. Steiner, *The Children's Cause* (Washington, D.C.: The Brookings Institution, 1976), p. 5.

65. Kenneth Keniston and the Carnegie Council for Children, *All Our Children: The American Family Under Pressure* (New York: Harcourt Brace Jovanovich, 1977), p. 18. See also pp. 3–23 for a description of the shift in authority.

66. *Ibid.*, and the National Academy of Sciences, Advisory Committee on Child Development, Assembly of Behavioral and Social Sciences, and National Research Council, *Toward a National Policy for Children and Families* (Washington, D.C.: National Academy of Sciences, 1976). The latter report also emphasized how the shifting style of the family to one parent, and/or working parent families, had placed a burden on child care.

67. C. Arden Miller, "Health Care of Children and Youth in America," *American Journal of Public Health* 65 (April 1975): 356.

68. Henry Dietrich, "For the Welfare of Children," Presidential Address, in American Academy of Pediatrics, *For the Welfare of Children* (Springfield, Ill.: Charles C. Thomas, 1955), p. 77.

69. Special Committee on the EMIC Program, *Journal of Pediatrics* 25 (1944): 91.

70. Warren R. Sisson, Presidential Address, 1950, in AAP, *For the Welfare of Children*, p. 218. The Children's Bureau at the time was proposing some public programs without a means test. The Academy was opposed to any programs except for those who could not afford to pay.

71. Warren Magnuson, as cited in U.S. Congress, Senate, Committee on Government Operations, Subcommittee on Executive Reorganization and Government Research, *Report: Federal Role in Health*, 91st Cong., 2d sess., 30 April 1970, p. 3.

72. Steiner argues that the Children's Bureau was in decline for some time before

its splintering in 1969. *The Children's Cause*, pp. 36–46. Whatever the case, the American Academy of Pediatrics and organized medicine as a whole had long been anxious for its demise.

73. American Academy of Pediatrics, Committee on School Health, *School Health: A Guide for Health Professionals* (Evanston, Ill.: American Academy of Pediatrics, 1977), p. 5. See also p. 2 of the 1972 edition of the same book, entitled *School Health: A Guide for Physicians*.

74. On misclassification and labeling, see Jane Mercer, "Discussion of Alternative Value Frames for Classification of Exceptional Children," paper prepared for the National Advisory Committee on Classification of Exceptional Children, Riverside, Calif., 1972. On educators prescribing for hyperactive children, see Judith M. Egert, "Now School Teachers are Playing Doctor," *Medical Economics*, 17 April 1978, pp. 119–24.

75. See, for example, the Robert Wood Johnson Foundation report on the school health programs it has supported in communities with large numbers of low-income children, *Special Report: School Health Services* (Princeton, N.J.: Robert Wood Johnson Foundation, 1979); and Philip R. Nader, ed., *Options for School Health: Meeting Community Needs* (Germantown, Md.: Aspen, 1978).

76. American Academy of Pediatrics, *Standards of Child Health Care* (Evanston, Ill.: American Academy of Pediatrics, 1967), unpaginated introduction.

77. AAP, *Lengthening Shadows*, p. 222. See also I. Barry Pless, "The Changing Face of Primary Pediatrics," *Pediatric Clinics of North America* 21 (February 1974): 223–44.

78. See, for example, the exchange of comments between Robert Haggerty, supporting the position that both family physicians and pediatricians were here to stay, each group with similar goals ("Family Medicine and Pediatrics," *American Journal of Diseases of Children* 126 [1973]: 13–14), and Hugh Thompson's reply, asserting the superiority of pediatricians in caring for children ("Letter: Family Medicine and Pediatrics, Reply to Robert Haggerty," *American Journal of Diseases of Children* 127 [April 1974]: 596).

79. This book has remained a best-seller for over sixty years. New editions every five to ten years have updated the information.

80. See Eliot, "Emergency Food Relief and Child Health," pp. 1–10, as cited in Bremner, ed., *Children and Youth*, 2:1083–88. Dr. Eliot had earlier undertaken a study on control of rickets, under the sponsorship of the Children's Bureau.

81. Josephine S. Baker, *Fighting for Life*, pp. 82–87, as cited in Bremner, ed., *Children and Youth*, 2:1060.

82. Haven Emerson, *Local Health Units for the Nation* (New York: Commonwealth Fund, 1945).

83. See the excellent case study of this program by Nathan Sinai and Odin Andersen, *EMIC: A Study of Administrative Experience* (Ann Arbor: University of Michigan Press, 1948). The hospitals and physicians were not always gracious about the bureau's standards-setting activities.

84. See L. Emmet Holt, *Diseases of Infancy and Childhood* (New York: Appleton and Co., 1897), pp. 122–237; and Thomas Morgan Rotch, *Pediatrics* (New York: Lippincott, 1901), pp. 112–245.

85. See L. Emmett Holt, John Howland, and Rustin McIntosh, *Holt's Diseases of Infancy and Childhood*, 10th ed. (New York: Appleton and Co., 1933); and Wilburt C. Davison, *The Compleat Pediatrician* (Durham, N.C.: Duke University Press,

1934), chap. III. However, this section was omitted from the 1938 and later editions.

86. Anne-Marie Foltz, "The Politics of Prevention: Child Health under Medicaid" (Ph.D. dissertation, Yale University, 1980), table C-3, pp. 363–370.

87. Henry L. K. Shaw, "The American Pediatric Society and Preventive Pediatrics," *American Journal of Diseases of Children* 38 (July 1929): 1.

88. Martha Clifford, "Better Health Examinations at Well-Child Conferences and Summer Round-Ups," *Connecticut Health Bulletin* 61 (February 1947): 43–45.

89. The Academy of Pediatrics had been formed out of a dissident group which had earlier supported the Sheppard-Towner Act of 1922, when the American Medical Association House of Delegates denounced it.

90. In 1938 the first academy book was the *Committee Report on Infectious Diseases* (the "Red Book"). Eighteen editions were published between 1938 and 1977, with 180,000 copies printed between 1966 and 1977. Among other publications were: *Standards and Recommendations for Hospital Care of Newborn Infants* (6 editions); *Standards of Child Health Care* (3 editions with 78,000 copies printed between 1967 and 1977); and *School Health: A Guide for Health Professionals* (2 editions).

91. See Charles E. Osborne and Hugh C. Thompson, "Criteria for Evaluation of Ambulatory Child Health Care by Chart Audit: Development and Testing of a Methodology," *Pediatrics* 56 (October 1975 supplement): 625–92.

92. See, for example, C. M. Allen and H. R. Shinefield, "Pediatric Multiphasic Program," *American Journal of Diseases of Children* 118 (September 1969): 469–72; Anderson, "Evaluation of Physical Examination in Infants"; Hoekelman, "What Constitutes Adequate Well-Baby Care?", pp. 313–26; Kessner, *Assessment of Medical Care*; A. H. McFarlane and G. R. Norman, "A Medical Care Information System: Evaluation of Changing Patterns of Primary Care," *Medical Care* 10 (June 1972): 481–87; Barbara Starfield *et al.*, "How 'Regular' is the 'Regular Source' of Medical Care?", *Pediatrics* 51 (May 1973): 822–32; and H. Steiner, "An Evaluation of Child Health Clinic Services in Newcastle-upon-Tyne during 1972–1974," *British Journal of Preventive and Social Medicine* 31 (March 1977): 1–5.

93. Joint Committee on Health Problems in Education, *Health Appraisal of School Children* (Washington, D.C.: National Education Association, 1969).

94. The three recommended schedules are listed in appendix II of John E. Fogarty International Center Task Force, *Preventive Medicine, USA: Theory, Practice, and Application of Prevention in Personal Health Services* (New York: Prodist, 1976).

95. U.S. Department of Health, Education, and Welfare, National Center for Health Statistics, "Ambulatory Medical Care Rendered in Pediatricians' Offices, 1975," Advance Data No. 12 (13 October 1977), fig. 2; and Starfield *et al.*, "How 'Regular' is the 'Regular Source'?", p. 823.

96. C. Henry Kempe, Remarks in Eli H. Newberger, ed., *Child Advocacy and Pediatrics: Report of the Eighth Ross Roundtable on Critical Approaches to Common Pediatric Problems* (Columbus, Ohio: Ross Laboratories, 1978), p. 50.

97. *Ibid.*

98. See, for example, the American Association for the Advancement of Science Working Group's report on Comprehensive Screening Services, which stated that only two screening programs had been found efficacious: mammography for women over fifty, and multiphasic screening in a health maintenance organization. The screening of children was among the topics considered but no efficacious

techniques could be verified on the basis of present knowledge. "Report from the Workshop on Health and Human Services Innovations," July 1979.

99. Foltz, "Politics of Prevention," table C-1, p. 358.

100. Henry James Parish, *A History of Immunization* (Edinburgh: Livingstone, 1965), pp. 1–2, 20–32.

101. Hugh Paul, *The Control of Communicable Diseases* (London: Harvey and Blythe, 1952), p. 68.

102. Geoffrey Edsall, "Efficacy of Immunization Procedures Used in Public Health Practice," in World Health Organization, *The Role of Immunization in Communicable Disease Control* (Public Health Paper No. 8), as reprinted by the U.S. Department of Health, Education, and Welfare, for distribution in the CDC seminar on immunization, 1963. Unpaginated.

103. "It is the imperative duty of a physician to see to it that every young infant is vaccinated. . . ." L. Emmet Holt, *The Diseases of Infancy and Childhood* (New York: Appleton and Co., 1897), p. 931. The same statement appears in the book's 9th ed. (1926) by L. Emmet Holt, Jr., and John Howland, p. 832.

104. John J. Hanlon, *Principles of Public Health Administration* (St. Louis: C. V. Mosby, 1964), p. 554.

105. Charles L. Jackson, "State Laws on Compulsory Immunization in the United States," *Public Health Reports* 84 (September 1969): 794.

106. National Immunization Work Group on Consent, "Report and Recommendations," *Report and Recommendations of the National Immunization Work Groups*, submitted to the Office of the Assistant Secretary for Health (McLean, Va.: JRB Associates, 1977), appendix A-1.

107. In England, whereas at least 70 percent of infants were vaccinated between 1850 and 1900, only 34 percent were vaccinated in 1939. Parish, *History of Immunization*, pp. 30, 34.

108. Jackson, "State Laws on Immunization," p. 794.

109. John E. Gordon, *Control of Communicable Diseases in Man* (New York: American Public Health Association, 1965), pp. 2–3. Twelve editions were published between 1917 and 1975.

110. Of the pediatric textbooks surveyed (see appendix 2 of the present work) all but one which cited a reference for immunization schedules cited the AAP Red Book. For example, "The Pediatric Red Book is the best reference for adopting an immunization program and should be followed." Lee W. Bass and Jerome H. Wolfson, *The Style and Management of Pediatric Practice* (Pittsburgh: University of Pittsburgh Press, 1977), p. 64. "Best known and authoritative in this [immunization] field is the Red Book of the Academy of Pediatrics." Edward B. Shaw and Moses Grossman, "Active Immunization—Infectious Diseases," in Harry Cameron Shirkey, ed., *Pediatric Therapy*, 4th ed. (St. Louis: C. V. Mosby, 1972), p. 369.

111. For its formation and early history, see Ralph C. Williams, *The United States Public Health Service, 1798–1950* (Washington, D.C.: Commissioned Officers Association of the U.S. Public Health Service, 1951), pp. 396–403.

112. U.S. Congress, House, *Report from the Committee on Interstate and Foreign Commerce to Accompany H.R. 10541*, 87th Cong., 2d sess., 18 June 1962, pp. 3, 5.

113. Shaw and Grossman, "Active Immunization," p. 369.

114. American Academy of Pediatrics, *Report of the Committee on Infectious Diseases*, 18th ed. (Evanston, Ill.: American Academy of Pediatrics, 1977), p. 2.

115. Shirley L. Fannin, "Immunization Practice" in Sidney S. Gellis and Benjamin Kagan, *Current Pediatric Therapy*, 8th ed. (Philadelphia: W. B. Saunders, 1978), p. 668.

116. U.S. Congress, House, *Report to Accompany H.R. 10541*, pp. 3, 5; National Immunization Work Group on Policy, *Reports and Recommendations of the National Immunization Groups* (McLean, Va.: JRB Associates, 1977), table 1.

117. U.S. Department of Health, Education, and Welfare, *Summary of Immunization Status for Polio, DTP, Measles, Rubella and Mumps, 1977*, Preliminary Report (Atlanta, Ga.: Center for Disease Control, 1977), p. 2.

118. *Ibid.*, p. 3.

119. See U.S. Department of Health, Education, and Welfare, *Immunizations Survey*, for the years 1967 to 1977.

120. David B. McDaniel, Edward W. Patton, and John A. Mather, "Immunization Activities of Private Practice Physicians: A Record Audit," *Pediatrics* 56 (October 1975): 506.

121. *Ibid.*, p. 504.

122. Edgar K. Marcuse, "Commentaries: Immunization: An Embarrassing Failure," *Pediatrics* 56 (October 1975): 493.

123. *Ibid.*, p. 494.

124. "Experts' interviews said that everyone must share the blame for the apathy. Dr. Charles R. Webb, Jr., the Texas Health Department epidemiologist, said, 'Kids don't like to get shots. Busy parents are loathe to take time off from work or bowling to fight their kids to get shots.' To Dr. James Chin, the California State Health Department epidemiologist, the low immunization levels reflect 'professional and public apathy.'" Lawrence K. Altman, "Low Immunization Figures are Attributed to Apathy of Public, Health Professionals, and Government Aides," *New York Times*, 7 April 1977, p. A14.

125. See below for a discussion of the rubella controversy, which may be the one exception.

126. P. D. Hooper, "Letter: Developmental Screening and Assessment," *British Medical Journal* 2 (12 April 1975): 87.

127. See n. 6 to chap. 6, giving references for screening.

128. *Crisis in Child Mental Health: Challenge for the 1970's* (New York: Harper and Row, 1970), p. 38.

129. James S. Kakalik, Garry D. Brewer, *et al.*, *Services for Handicapped Youth: A Program Overview* (Santa Monica, Calif.: Rand, 1973), p. 274.

130. William K. Frankenburg and A. Frederick North, *A Guide to Screening for the Early and Periodic Screening, Diagnosis, and Treatment Program under Medicaid* (Washington, D.C.: Social and Rehabilitation Service, Department of Health, Education, and Welfare, 1974), p. 141.

131. J. R. Metz, C. M. Allen, *et al.*, "A Pediatric Screening Examination for Psychosocial Problems," *Pediatrics* 58 (October 1976): 595–606.

132. *Standards for Child Health Care*, 1972 and 1977.

133. Frankenburg and North, *A Guide to Screening*, pp. 142–44.

134. U.S. Department of Health, Education, and Welfare, Medical Services Administration, unpublished report on developmental assessment, 1976.

135. W. K. Frankenburg, W. J. Van Doorninck, *et al.*, "The Denver Prescreening Developmental Questionnaire," *Pediatrics* 57 (May 1976): 744–53.

136. W. K. Frankenburg, N. P. Dick, and J. Darland, "Development of Pre-School Aged Children of Different Social and Ethnic Groups: Implications for Developmental Screening," *Journal of Pediatrics* 87 (July 1975): 125–32.

137. See, for example, "Developmental Screening" (Editorial), *Lancet* 1 (5 April 1975): 784–86.

138. "Developmental Assessment in EPSDT," *American Journal of Orthopsychiatry* 48 (January 1978): 16.

139. *Developmental Review in the EPSDT Program* (Washington, D.C.: U.S. Department of Health, Education, and Welfare, 1977), p. xiii.

140. *EPSDT: Does it Spell Health Care for Poor Children?* (Washington, D.C.: Children's Defense Fund, 1977), p. 180.

141. *Ibid.*

142. A Frederick North, Jr., "Screening in Child Health Care: Where Are We Now and Where Are We Going?", *Pediatrics* 54 (November 1974): 632.

143. K. S. Holt, "Screening for Disease: Infancy and Childhood," *Lancet* 2 (2 November 1974): 1057.

144. David S. Mundel, "Policy for Primary Medical Care for Children: A Framework of Basic Choices," in Harvard Child Health Project, vol. 3: *Developing a Better Health Care System for Children* (Cambridge, Mass.: Ballinger, 1977), p. 17.

145. This high number of recommended visits may also be an artifact of sampling that was restricted by the availability of books from this period. Three major pediatric textbooks were identified for the period. Of these, only two were sampled, each for one edition only. (See appendix 2 of the present work for pediatric books reviewed.)

146. "Commentary: Child Health Supervision—Is It Worth It?", *Pediatrics* 52 (August 1973): 273.

147. Robert M. Heavenrich, "Child Health Supervision—Is It Worth It? A Response," *Pediatrics* 52 (August 1973): 278.

148. Robert W. Chamberlin, "Letter," *Pediatrics* 53 (March 1974): 445–46.

149. Page 12.

150. R. L. Mindlin and P. M. Densen, "Medical Care of Urban Infants: Health Supervision," *American Journal of Public Health* 61 (1971): 687–97.

151. Barbara Starfield, Henry Seidel, *et al.*, "Private Pediatric Practice: Performance and Problems," *Pediatrics* 52 (September 1973): 344–51.

152. Gunnar B. Stickler, "How Necessary is the Routine Check-up?" *Clinical Pediatrics* 6 (1967): 454.

153. C. M. Allen and H. R. Shinefield, "Automatic Multiphasic Screening, " *Pediatrics* 54 (1974): 621.

Chapter 7

154. The account that follows is based mainly on the following sources: Philip M. Boffey, "Anatomy of a Decision: How the Nation Declared War on Swine Flu," *Science* 192 (14 May 1976): 63–41; and Richard E. Neustadt and Harvey V. Fineberg, *The Swine Flu Affair: Decision-Making on a Slippery Disease* (Washington, D.C.: Government Printing Office, 1978). See also U.S. Comptroller General, *The Swine Flu*

Program: An Unprecedented Venture into Preventive Medicine, HRD 77-115 (Washington, D.C.: General Accounting Office, 1977).

155. On 4 March 1978, p. 34. Rubella is German measles.

156. "[It is] more than undemocratic to allow state agencies to unilaterally coerce reputable physicians to condone medical procedures with their patients which the physician deems unreliable." Dr. Albert Peacock, Record of the Hearings of the Committee on Public Health and Safety, Connecticut State Legislature, 3 March 1978, p. 21.

157. *Ibid.*, p. 26, and Richard Quintiliani, *ibid.*, p. 30. Dr. Peacock went on to point out other programs recommended by these organizations which had failed, and Dr. Quintiliani continued about the swine flu program that " . . . there's several billions of dollars in lawsuits over adverse effects relating to a vaccine that was supported by all the supposed committees" (p. 30).

158. John Lewis, *ibid.*, p. 59.

159. Robert Harris, *ibid.*, p. 67.

160. Representative Chester W. Morgan, *ibid.*, p. 62.

161. Among the ties between the opponents of rubella immunization and the committee members were: one of the physicians was a constituent of one of the committee members and was well known to him; one of the physicians had recently successfully diagnosed a case of hepatitis in another committee member, a case which had gone undiagnosed for six months by other physicians. Stephanie Cameron, interview, 21 March 1978.

162. Public Act No. 78-165, Connecticut State Legislature.

163. U.S. Department of Health, Education, and Welfare, *Early and Periodic Screening, Diagnosis, and Treatment*, Medical Services Administration, PRG 21 (28 June 1972). The procedures recommended were: health and developmental history; physical growth and developmental assessment; unclothed physical inspection; ear, nose, mouth, and throat inspection; vision and hearing testing; tests for anemia, sickle cell, and tuberculosis; urine and lead poisoning screening; and assessment of nutritional and immunization status.

164. These states were Kentucky, Oklahoma, Texas, Iowa, Kansas, Missouri, Nebraska, and Montana. See table 9 for the note about Texas.

165. Frankenburg and North, *A Guide to Screening*, 1974.

166. Anne-Marie Foltz and Donna Brown, "State Response to Federal Policy: Children, EPSDT, and the Medicaid Muddle," *Medical Care* 13 (August 1975): 640.

167. Hal L. Harle, M.D., interview, 22 February 1978.

168. Duncan Neuhauser, "The Public Voice and the Nation's Health," *Milbank Memorial Fund Quarterly/Health and Society* 57 (Winter 1979): 68.

Conclusion

1. Seymour Perry and John T. Kalberer, Jr., "Special Report: The NIH Consensus-Development Program and the Assessment of Health Care Technologies: The First Two Years," *New England Journal of Medicine* 303 (17 July 1980): 169–72.

2. The question was whether women should be screened for cervical cancer annually or every three years. Fran Pollner, "NIH Panelists Compromise on Pap Smear," *Medical News*, 22 September 1980, pp. 1, 5.

3. Gilbert Steiner, *The Children's Cause* (Washington, D.C.: Brookings Institution, 1976), pp. 221–31.

4. Martha Derthick, "No More Easy Votes for Social Security," *Brookings Bulletin* 16 (Fall 1979): 1–5.

5. Ian Lustick, "Explaining the Variable Utility of Disjointed Incrementalism: Four Propositions," *American Political Science Review* 74 (June 1980): 342–53.

Bibliography

General

Books and Articles

Allen, C. M., and Shinefield, H. R. "Automated Multiphasic Screening." *Pediatrics* 54 (1974): 621–26.

———— "Pediatric Multiphasic Program." *Amercian Journal of Diseases of Children* 118 (September 1969): 469–72.

Allison, Graham T. "Conceptual Models and the Cuban Missile Crisis." *American Political Science Review* 63 (September 1969): 689–718.

Alpert, Joel J.; Heagerty, Margaret; Robertson, Leon; Kosa, John; and Haggerty, Robert J. "Effective Use of Comprehensive Pediatric Care." *American Journal of Diseases of Children* 116 (November 1968): 529–33.

Alpert, Joel J.; Robertson, Leon S.; Kosa, John; Heagarty, Margaret C.; and Haggerty, Robert J. "Delivery of Health Care for Children: Report of An Experiment." *Pediatrics* 57 (June 1976): 917–30.

Altenstetter, Christa, and Bjorkman, James Warner. *Federal-State Health Policies and Impacts: The Politics of Implementation.* Washington, D.C.: University Press of America, 1978.

Altman, Lawrence K. "Low Immunization Figures are Attributed to Apathy of Public, Health Professionals, and Government Aides." *New York Times*, 7 April 1977.

American Academy of Pediatrics. *Child Health Services and Pediatric Education: Report of the Committee for the Study of Child Health Services.* New York: Commonwealth Fund, 1949.

———— *For the Welfare of Children.* Springfield, Ill.: Charles C. Thomas, 1955.

———— *Lengthening Shadows: A Report of the Council on Pediatric Practice.* Evanston, Ill.: American Academy of Pediatrics, 1970.

American Medical Association. *Distribution of Physicians, Hospitals and Hospital Beds in the U.S., 1972,* I. Chicago: American Medical Association, 1972.

American Public Health Association. "Policy Statement: The State Public Health Agency." *American Journal of Public Health* 55 (December 1965): 2011–20.

American Public Welfare Association. "Essentials of Public Welfare: A Statement of Principles." *Public Welfare* 11 (January 1953): 3.

Anderson, F. P. "Evaluation of the Routine Physical Examination of Infants in the First Year of Life." *Pediatrics* 45 (1970): 950–60.

Avery, Allyson Davies; Lelah, Tova; Solomon, Nancy E.; Harris, L. Jeff; Brook, Robert H.; Greenfield, Sheldon; Ware, John E.; and Avery, Charles H. *Quality of Medical Care Assessment Using Outcome Measures: Eight Disease-Specific Applications.* Santa Monica, Calif.: Rand, 1976.

Bardach, Eugene. *The Implementation Game: What Happens After a Bill Becomes a Law.* Cambridge, Mass.: MIT Press, 1977.

Bergman, Abraham B. "The Menace of Mass Screening" (editorial). *American Journal of Public Health* 67 (June 1977): 601–2.

Blake, John B. *Origins of Maternal and Child Health Programs*. New Haven: Yale School of Medicine, 1953.

Boffey, Philip M. "Anatomy of a Decision: How the Nation Declared War on Swine Flu." *Science* 192 (May 1976): 636–41.

Bradbury, Dorothy E. *Five Decades of Action for Children: A History of the Children's Bureau*. Washington, D.C.: Department of Health, Education, and Welfare, 1962.

Bremner, Robert H., ed. *Children and Youth in America: A Documentary History*. 3 vols. Cambridge, Mass.: Harvard University Press, 1970–74.

Breslow, Lester, and Somers, Anne R. "The Lifetime Health-Monitoring Program." *New England Journal of Medicine* 296 (March 1977): 602–3.

Brook, Robert H. "Quality of Care Assessment: Policy Relevant Issues." *Policy Sciences* 5 (1974): 317–41.

Buntz, C. Gregory; Macaluso, Theodore F.; and Azarow, Jay Allen. "Federal Influence on State Health Policy." *Journal of Health Politics, Policy and Law* 3 (Spring 1978): 71–86.

Chamberlin, Robert W. "Letter." *Pediatrics* 53 (March 1974): 445–46.

Clifford, Martha. "Better Health Examinations at Well-Child Conferences and Summer Round-Ups." *Connecticut Health Bulletin* 61 (February 1947): 43–45.

Cochrane, A. L. *Effectiveness and Efficiency*. London: Oxford University Press for Nuffield Provincial Hospitals Trust, 1972.

——— "The History of the Measurement of Ill Health." *International Journal of Epidemiology* 1 (1972): 89–92.

Cochrane, A. L., and Holland, W. W. "Validation of Screening Procedures." *British Medical Bulletin* 27 (1971): 3–8.

Collen, Morris F. "A Case Study of Multiphasic Health Testing." In National Academy of Sciences, *Medical Technology and the Health Care System: A Study of Equipment Embodied Technology*, pp. 124–72. Report by the Committee on Technology and Health Care, Assembly of Engineering, National Research Council and Institute of Medicine. Washington, D.C.: National Academy of Sciences, 1978.

——— "Periodic Health Examinations: Why? What? When? How?" *Primary Care* 3 (1976): 201.

Commission on Chronic Illness. *Chronic Illness in the United States*, I. Cambridge, Mass.: Harvard University Press, 1957.

Committee on the Cost of Medical Care. *Medical Care for the American People: The Final Report*. Chicago: University of Chicago Press, 1932; reprint ed., Washington, D.C.: U.S. Health Services and Mental Health Administration, Community Health Service, 1970.

Cooper, Barbara S., and McGee, Mary F. "Medical Care Outlays for Three Age Groups: Young, Intermediate, and Aged." *Social Security Bulletin* 34 (May 1971): 3–14.

Cooper, Barbara S.; Worthington, Nancy L.; and Prio, Paula A. "National Health Expenditures, 1929–73." *Social Security Bulletin* 37 (February 1974): 3–19, 48.

Davis, Karen. "Hospital Costs and the Medicare Program." *Social Security Bulletin* 36 (August 1973): 18–36.

Davis, Karen, and Schoen, Cathy. *Health and the War on Poverty: A Ten-Year Ap-

praisal. Washington, D.C.: Brookings Institution, 1978.

De Geyndt, Willy. "Organization and Delivery of Comprehensive Health Services with Major Emphasis on Services to Children and on the Role of the Federal Government." Ph.D. dissertation, University of Minnesota, 1970.

DelBlanco, Thomas L. "The Periodic Health Examination for the Adult: Waste or Wisdom." *Primary Care* 3 (June 1976): 205–14.

Derthick, Martha. *The Influence of Federal Grants*. Cambridge, Mass.: Harvard University Press, 1970.

———— *New Towns In-Town*. Washington, D.C.: Urban Institute, 1972.

De Tocqueville, Alexis. *Democracy in America*, I. New York: Vintage Books, 1955.

Downs, Anthony. *Inside Bureaucracy*. Boston: Little, Brown, 1967.

Dubos, Rene. *Mirage of Health*. New York: Harper and Row, 1959.

Egert, Judith M. "Now School Teachers are Playing Doctor." *Medical Economics*, 17 April 1978, pp. 119–24.

Elsom, Kendall A.; Spoont, Stanley; and Potter, H. Phelps. "An Appraisal of the Periodic Health Examination." *Industrial Medicine and Surgery* 25 (August 1956): 367–71.

Emerson, Haven. *Local Health Units for the Nation*. New York: Commonwealth Fund, 1945.

Etzioni, Amitai. *Genetic Fix*. New York: Harper and Row, 1973.

Fannin, Shirley L. "Immunization Practice." In Sidney S. Gellis and Benjamin Kagan, *Current Pediatric Therapy*, pp. 668–74. 8th ed. Philadelphia: W. B. Saunders, 1978.

Foltz, Anne-Marie, and Kelsey, Jennifer L. "The Annual Pap Test: A Dubious Policy Success." *Milbank Memorial Fund Quarterly/Health and Society* 56 (Fall 1978): 426–62.

Franco, S. Charles. "The Early Detection of Disease by Periodic Examination." *Industrial Medicine and Surgery* 25 (June 1956): 251–57.

Frankenburg, W. K.; Dick, N. P.; and Darland, J. "Development of Pre-School Aged Children of Different Social and Ethnic Groups: Implications for Developmental Screening." *Journal of Pediatrics* 87 (July 1975): 125–32.

Frankenburg, W. K.; Van Doorninck, W. J.; Liddell, Theresa; and Dick, Nathan P. "The Denver Prescreening Developmental Questionnaire (PDQ)." *Pediatrics* 57 (May 1976): 744–53.

Freymann, John Gordon. "Medicine's Great Schism: Prevention vs. Cure: An Historical Interpretation." *Medical Care* 13 (July 1975): 525–36.

Galdston, Iago. "The Genealogy of the Health Examination." *The Health Examiner* 1 (February 1932): 7–14.

Gibson, R. M., and Fisher, C. R. "National Health Expenditures, Fiscal Year 1977." *Social Security Bulletin* 4 (July 1976): 3–20.

Ginzberg, Eli, and Solow, Robert M., eds. *The Great Society: Lessons for the Future*. New York: Basic Books, 1974.

Golden, Archie S. *An Inventory for Primary Health Care Practice*. Cambridge, Mass.: Ballinger, 1976.

Gordis, Leon. "Effectiveness of Comprehensive Care Programs in Preventing Rheumatic Fever." *New England Journal of Medicine* 289 (August 1973): 372–73.

Gordis, Leon, and Markowitz, Milton. "Evaluation of the Effectiveness of Comprehensive and Continuous Pediatric Care." *Pediatrics* 48 (November 1971): 766–76.

Gordon, John E. *Control of Communicable Diseases in Man.* New York: American Public Health Association, 1965.

Haar, Charles M. *Between the Idea and the Reality: A Study in the Origin, Fate and Legacy of the Model Cities Program.* Boston: Little, Brown, 1975.

Haggerty, Robert. "Family Medicine and Pediatrics." *American Journal of Diseases of Children* 126 (1973): 13–14.

Hansen, Holger. "Prevention of Mental Retardation Due to PKU: Selected Aspects of Program Validity." *Preventive Medicine* 4 (1975): 310–21.

Hansen, M. F., and Aradine, Carolyn. "The Changing Face of Primary Pediatrics: Review and Commentary." *Pediatric Clinics of North America* 21 (February 1974): 245–56.

Hargrove, Erwin C. *The Missing Link: The Study of the Implementation of Social Policy.* Washington, D.C.: Urban Institute, 1975.

Harnes, Jack R. "Second and Subsequent Periodic Examinations." *New York State Journal of Medicine* 76 (June 1976): 891–97.

Hart, Cyril J. R., ed. *Screening in General Practice.* Edinburgh: Churchill Livingstone, 1975.

Harvard Child Health Project. Vol. 1: *Toward a Primary Medical Care System Responsive to Children's Needs.* Vol. 2: *Children's Medical Care Needs and Treatment.* Vol. 3: *Developing a Better Health Care System for Children.* Cambridge, Mass.: Ballinger, 1977.

Heavenrich, Robert M. "Child Health Supervision—Is It Worth It? A Response." *Pediatrics* 52 (August 1973): 278.

Hoekelman, Robert A. "What Constitutes Adequate Well-baby Care?" *Pediatrics* 55 (March 1975): 313–26.

Holahan, John; Scanlon, William; and Spitz, Bruce. *Restructuring Federal Medicaid Controls and Incentives.* Washington, D.C.: Urban Institute, 1977.

Holland, W. W. "Screening: Taking Stock." *Lancet* 2 (December 1974): 1494–96.

Holt, K. S. "Screening for Disease: Infancy and Childhood." *Lancet* 2 (November 1974): 1057–60.

Hooper, P. D. "Letter: Developmental Screening and Assessment." *British Medical Journal* 2 (April 1975): 87.

Iglehart, John K. "Health Report/HEW Plans to Fine States for Not Implementing Program." *National Journal,* 11 January 1975, pp. 59–61.

Ingraham, Elizabeth A. "Connecticut Need for Child Hygiene Work." *Connecticut Health Bulletin* 40 (May 1926): 115–18.

Institute of Medicine. *Interim Report of a Study: Primary Care in Medicine: A Definition.* Washington, D.C.: National Academy of Sciences, 1977.

Jackson, Charles L. "State Laws on Compulsory Immunization in the United States." *Public Health Reports* 84 (September 1969): 788–95.

John E. Fogarty International Center Task Force. *Preventive Medicine, USA: Theory, Practice, and Application of Prevention in Personal Health Services.* New York: Prodist, 1976.

Joint Commission on the Mental Health of Children. *Crisis in Child Mental Health:*

Challenge for the 1970's. New York: Harper and Row, 1970.

Joint Committee on Health Problems in Education. *Health Appraisal of School Children*. Washington, D.C.: National Education Association, 1969.

Kakalik, James S.; Brewer, Garry D.; Dougharty, Laurence A.; Fleischauer, Patricia D.; and Genensky, Samuel M. *Services for Handicapped Youth; A Program Overview*. Santa Monica, Calif.: Rand, 1973.

Keniston, Kenneth, and the Carnegie Council for Children. *All Our Children: The American Family Under Pressure*. New York: Harcourt Brace Jovanovich, 1977.

Kessner, David; Show, Carolyn Kalk; and Singer, James. *Assessment of Medical Care for Children*. Washington, D.C.: Institute of Medicine, National Academy of Sciences, 1974.

Korsch, Barbara M.; Negrete, Vida F.; Mercer, Ann S.; and Freeman, Barbara. "How Comprehensive Are Well Child Visits?" *American Journal of Diseases of Children* 112 (December 1971): 483–88.

Kramer, Michael S. "My Turn: The Risks of Health." *Newsweek*, 6 February 1978, p. 11.

Kugajevoky, Victor, and Lazar, Allan. "Controlling Eligibility Errors in the Medicaid Program." *Journal for Medicaid Management* 1 (Summer 1977): 7–13.

Lappe, Marc, *et al.* "Ethical and Social Issues in Screening for Genetic Disease." *New England Journal of Medicine* 286 (May 1972): 1129–32.

Lasswell, Harold D. *Politics: Who Gets What, When, How*. New York: P. Smith, 1959.

Levin, Arthur L. "Cost-Effectiveness in Maternal and Child Health: Implications for Program Planning and Evaluation." *New England Journal of Medicine* 278 (May 1968): 1041–47.

Lewis, Charles. "Does Comprehensive Care Make a Difference?" *American Journal of Diseases of Children* 122 (December 1971): 469–74.

Lindblom, Charles E. *The Intelligence of Democracy*. New York: The Free Press, 1965.

——— "The Science of Muddling Through." *Public Administration Review* 29 (Spring 1959): 79–88.

Lippard, Vernon. *The Crippled Child in New York City*. New York: Commission for the Study of Crippled Children, 1940.

Lustick, Ian. "Explaining the Variable Utility of Disjointed Incrementalism: Four Propositions." *American Political Science Review* 74 (June 1980): 342–53.

McDaniel, David B.; Patton, Edward W.; and Mather, John A. "Immunization Activities of Private Practice Physicians: A Record Audit." *Pediatrics* 56 (October 1975): 504–7.

McFarlane, A. H., and Norman, G. R. "A Medical Care Information System: Evaluation of Changing Patterns of Primary Care." *Medical Care* 10 (June 1972): 481–87.

McKeown, Thomas. "Validation of Screening Procedures." In Thomas McKeown, ed. *Screening in Medical Care: Reviewing the Evidence*, pp. 1–13. London: Oxford University Press, 1968.

Macrae, Norman. "America's Third Century." *The Economist*, 25–31 October 1975, Supplement.

Marcuse, Edgar K. "Commentaries: Immunization: An Embarrassing Failure." *Pediatrics* 56 (October 1975): 493–94.

Mayhew, David R. *Congress: The Electoral Connection.* New Haven: Yale University Press, 1974.

Mead, Lawrence M. *Institutional Analysis: An Approach to Implementation Problems in Medicaid.* Washington, D.C.: Urban Institute, 1977.

Mercer, Jane. "Discussion of Alternative Value Frames for Classification of Exceptional Children." Paper presented to the National Advisory Committee on Classification of Exceptional Children. Riverside, Calif., 1972.

Metz, J. R.; Allen, C. M.; Barr, George; and Shinefield, Henry. "A Pediatric Screening Examination for Psychosocial Problems." *Pediatrics* 58 (October 1976): 595–606.

Meyer, Ruben; Reuss, Joanne C.; Deniston, O. Lynn; Williams, George W.; and Chene, Douglas G. "Tracer Evaluation of Diagnosis and Treatment of EPSDT Referrals: Final Report: Executive Summary." University of Michigan School of Public Health, Ann Arbor, December 1976.

Miller, C. Arden. "Health Care of Children and Youth in America." *American Journal of Public Health* 65 (April 1975): 353–58.

Mindlin, R. L., and Densen, P. M. "Medical Care of Urban Infants: Health Supervision." *American Journal of Public Health* 61 (1971): 687–97.

Moynihan, Daniel P. *Maximum Feasible Misunderstanding.* New York: Free Press, 1969.

Mundel, David S. "Policy for Primary Medical Care for Children." Harvard Child Health Project, Vol. 3: *Developing a Better Health Care System for Children,* pp. 9–24. Cambridge, Mass.: Ballinger, 1977.

Murphy, Jerome T. *Grease the Squeaky Wheel: A Report on the Implementation of Title V of the Elementary and Secondary Education Act of 1965, Grants to Strengthen State Departments of Education.* Cambridge, Mass.: Center for Educational Policy Research, Harvard Graduate School of Education, 1973.

Nader, Philip R., ed. *Options for School Health: Meeting Community Needs.* Germantown, Md.: Aspen, 1978.

National Academy of Sciences, Advisory Committee on Child Development, Assembly of Behavioral and Social Sciences, and National Research Council. *Toward a National Policy for Children and Families.* Washington, D.C.: National Academy of Sciences, 1976.

National Council for Organizations for Children and Youth. *America's Children, 1976.* Washington, D.C.: National Council for Organizations for Children and Youth, 1976.

National Immunization Work Group on Consent. "Report and Recommendations." *Report and Recommendations of the National Immunization Work Groups.* Submitted to the Office of the Assistant Secretary for Health. McLean, Va.: JRB Associates, 1977.

Neuhauser, Duncan. "The Public Voice and the Nation's Health." *Milbank Memorial Fund Quarterly/Health and Society* 57 (Winter 1979): 60–69.

Newberger, Eli M., ed. *Child Advocacy and Pediatrics.* Report to the Eighth Ross Roundtable on Critical Approaches to Common Pediatric Problems in Collaboration with the Ambulatory Pediatric Association. Columbus, Ohio: Ross Laboratories, 1978.

New York Academy of Medicine. *Bulletin: Prevention and Health Maintenance Revisited; 1974 Annual Health Conference* 51 (January 1975).

North, A. Frederick, Jr. "Screening in Child Health Care: Where Are We Now and Where Are We Going?" *Pediatrics* 54 (November 1974): 631–40.

Osborne, Charles E., and Thompson, Hugh C. "Criteria for Evaluation of Ambulatory Child Health Care by Chart Audit: Development and Testing of a Methodology." *Pediatrics* 56 (October 1975 suppl.): 625–92.

Parish, Henry James. *History of Immunization*. Edinburgh: Livingstone, 1965.

Paul, Hugh. *The Control of Communicable Diseases*. London: Harvey and Blythe, 1952.

Perry, Seymour, and Kalberer, John T., Jr. "Special Report: The NIH Consensus-Development Program and the Assessment of Health Care Technologies: The First Two Years." *New England Journal of Medicine* 303 (July 1980): 169–72.

Pfaff, William. "Mr. Carter's Slide Rule." *New York Times*, 22 June 1979, p. A27.

Pless, I. Barry. "The Changing Face of Primary Pediatrics." *Pediatric Clinics of North America* 21 (February 1974): 223–44.

Pressman, Jeffrey L., and Wildavsky, Aaron B. *Implementation: How Great Expectations in Washington are Dashed in Oakland; Or Why It's Amazing that Federal Programs Work at All, This Being a Saga of the Economic Development Administration as Told by Two Sympathetic Observers Who Seek to Build Morals on a Foundation of Ruined Hopes*. Berkeley: University of California Press, 1973.

Robert Wood Johnson Foundation. *Special Report: School Health Services*. Princeton, N.J.: Robert Wood Johnson Foundation, 1979.

Rogers, David E. "The Challenge of Primary Care." *Daedalus: Doing Better and Feeling Worse: Health Care in the United States* 106 (Winter 1977): 81–103.

Rosen, George. *Preventive Medicine in the United States 1900–1975*. New York: Science History Publications, 1975.

Rosenbloom, Arlen L., and Ongley, James P. "Who Provides What Services to Children in Private Medical Practice?" *American Journal of Diseases of Children* 127 (March 1974): 357–61.

Sackett, David L., and Holland, W. W. "Controversy in the Detection of Disease." *Lancet* 2 (August 1975): 358–59.

Sanford, Terry. *Storm Over the States*. New York: McGraw Hill, 1967.

Sapolsky, Harvey. *The Polaris System Development: Bureaucratic Success in Government*. Cambridge, Mass.: Harvard University Press, 1972.

Schlesinger, Edward R. "The Sheppard-Towner Era: A Prototype Case Study in Federal-State Relationships." *American Journal of Public Health* 57 (1967): 1034–40.

Schonfeld, Hyman K.; Heston, Jean F.; and Falk, Isadore S. *Standards for Good Medical Care Based on the Opinions of Clinicians Associated with the Yale-New Haven Medical Center with Respect to 242 Diseases*. PB-240-385. Springfield, Va.: National Technical Information Service, 1975.

Schor, Stanley S., and Clark, Thomas W. "An Evaluation of the Periodic Health Examination: The Findings in 350 Examinees Who Died." *Annals of Internal Medicine* 61 (November 1964): 999–1005.

Seidman, Harold. *Politics, Position, and Power: The Dynamics of Federal Organization*. 2d ed. New York: Oxford University Press, 1975.

Sharp, C. L. E. H., and Keen, Harry, eds. *Presymptomatic Detection and Early Diagnosis: A Critical Appraisal*. London: Pittman, 1968.

Silver, George A. *Child Health: America's Future*. Germantown, Md.; Aspen, 1978.

————— *Politics and Social Policy: Failures in Child Health Services*. New Haven: Yale University Health Policy Project, 1976.

Simon, Herbert A. *Administrative Behavior: A Study of Decision-Making Processes in Administrative Organizations*. New York: The Free Press, 1957.

————— "On the Concept of Organizational Goals." In *A Sociological Reader on Complex Organizations*, pp. 158–74. Edited by Amitai Etzioni. New York: Holt, Rinehart and Winston, 1969.

Sinai, Nathan, and Anderson, Odin W. *EMIC: A Study of Administrative Experience*. Ann Arbor: University of Michigan Press, 1948.

Spark, Richard. "The Case Against Regular Physicals." *The New York Times Magazine*, 25 July 1976, pp. 10–11, 38–41.

Spitzer, Walter O., and Brown, Bruce P. "Unanswered Questions about the Periodic Health Examination." *Annals of Internal Medicine* 83 (1975): 257–63.

Starfield, Barbara. "Iron-Deficiency Anemia." Harvard Child Health Project, Vol. 2: *Children's Medical Care Needs and Treatment*, pp. 77–120. Cambridge, Mass.: Ballinger, 1977.

Starfield, Barbara; Bice, Thomas; Schach, Elizabeth; Rabin, David; and White, Kerr L. "How 'Regular' is the 'Regular Source' of Medical Care?" *Pediatrics* 51 (May 1973): 822–32.

Starfield, Barbara; Seidel, Henry; Carter, Gertrude; Garvin, William; and Seddon, Johanna. "Private Pediatric Practice: Performance and Problems." *Pediatrics* 52 121(September 1973): 344–51.

Steiner, Gilbert Y. *The Children's Cause*. Washington, D.C.: Brookings Institution, 1976.

————— *The State of Welfare*. Washington, D.C.: Brookings Institution, 1971.

Steiner, H. "An Evaluation of Child Health Clinic Services in Newcastle-upon-Tyne during 1972–1974." *British Journal of Preventive and Social Medicine* 31 (March 1977): 1–5.

Stevens, Robert B., and Stevens, Rosemary A. *Welfare Medicine in America*. New York: The Free Press, 1974.

Stevens, Rosemary. *American Medicine and the Public Interest*. New Haven: Yale University Press, 1971.

Stevens, Rosemary, and Stevens, Robert. "Medicaid: Anatomy of a Dilemma." *Law and Contemporary Problems: Health Care* 1 (Spring 1970): 365–78.

Stickler, Gunnar B. "How Necessary is the Routine Check-Up?" *Clinical Pediatrics* 6 (1967): 454.

Stuart, Bruce. "Equity and Medicaid." *Journal of Human Resources* 7 (Spring 1972): 162–78.

Sundquist, James L., and Davis, David W. *Making Federalism Work*. Washington, D.C.: Brookings Institution, 1969.

Thomas, Lewis. "On the Science and Technology of Medicine." *Daedalus* 106 (Winter 1977): 35–46.

Thompson, Charles E.; Zaus, Earl A.; and Keller, Philip R. "Some Observations on Periodic Health Examinations." *Journal of Occupational Medicine* 3 (April 1961): 215–17.

Thompson, Hugh. "Letter: Family Medicine and Pediatrics, Reply to Robert Haggerty." *American Journal of Diseases of Children* 127 (April 1974): 596.

———— "Preventive Services for Children." *Pediatric Clinics of North America* 16 (November 1969): 947–55.

Thorner, Robert M., and Crumpacker, E. L. "Mortality and Periodic Examinations of Executives." *Archives of Environmental Health* 3 (November 1961): 523–25.

Thorner, Robert M., and Remein, Q. R. *Principles and Procedures in the Evaluation of Screening for Disease.* Monograph #67. Washington, D.C.: Public Health Service, 1961.

Tyndall, Robert. "An Overview of the Texas Recipient Health Care Education Program." In *Patient and Provider Profiling (S/UR): Conference Summary,* pp. 238–43. Edited by Pacif Consultants. Washington, D.C.: U.S. Department of Health, Education, and Welfare, Institute for Medicaid Management, 1977.

Van Horn, A. L. "Crippled Children." *Social Work Year Book, 1947,* pp. 138–44. New York: Russell Sage Foundation, 1947.

Whitby, L. "Screening Definitions and Criteria." *Lancet* 2 (October 1974): 819–21.

Wholey, Joseph S. *The Absence of Program Evaluation as an Obstacle to Effective Public Expenditure Policy: A Case Study of Child Health Care Programs.* Washington, D.C.: Urban Institute, n.d.

Williams, Ralph C. *The United States Public Health Service, 1798–1950.* Washington, D.C.: Commissioned Officers Association of the U.S. Public Health Service, 1951.

Wilson, J. M. G., and Jungner, G. *Principles and Practices of Screening for Disease.* Public Health Paper #34. Geneva: World Health Organization, 1968.

Winston, Ellen. "Implications of the 1965 Amendments to the Social Security Act." *Social Work* 10 (October 1965): 10–15.

Witte, Edwin E. *The Development of the Social Security Act.* Madison: University of Wisconsin Press, 1963.

Wright, Deil S. *Understanding Intergovernmental Relations.* North Scituate, Mass.: Duxbury Press, 1978.

Yankauer, Alfred. "Commentary: Child Health Supervision—Is It Worth It?" *Pediatrics* 52 (August 1973): 273.

Yankauer, Alfred; Connelly, John P.; and Feldman, Jacob J. "Pediatric Practice in the United States with Special Attention to Utilization of Allied Health Workers." *Pediatrics* 45 (March 1970 suppl.).

Yankauer, Alfred, and Lawrence, Ruth. "A Study of Periodic School Medical Examinations: II. The Annual Increment of New Defects." *American Journal of Public Health* 46 (December 1556): 1953–62.

Government Documents

Advisory Commission on Intergovernmental Relations. *Categorical Grants: Their Role and Design.* Washington, D.C.: Government Printing Office, 1977.

———— *Intergovernmental Problems in Medicaid, A Commission Report.* September 1968.

———— *Statutory and Administrative Controls Associated with Federal Grants for Public Assistance.* Washington, D.C.: Advisory Commission on Intergovernmental Relations, 1964.

Connecticut Department of Finance and Control. *Digest of Administrative Reports to the Governor.* Hartford: Connecticut Department of Finance and Control, 1947–1979.

Connecticut Public Expenditure Council. *Connecticut State Revenues, Expenditures, Employees from 1950*. Hartford: Connecticut Public Expenditure Council, 1978.

Meyers, Samuel M., and McIntyre, Jennie. "Welfare Policy and Its Consequences for the Recipient Population: A Study of the AFDC Program." Report submitted to the U.S. Department of Health, Education, and Welfare, Social and Rehabilitation Service, December 1969.

Neustadt, Richard E., and Fineberg, Harvey V. *The Swine Flu Affair: Decision-Making on a Slippery Disease*. Washington, D.C.: Government Printing Office, 1978.

Report of Task Force on Medicaid Reform. Washington, D.C.: National Governors' Conference, 1977.

Task Force on Medicaid and Related Programs, Report. Washington, D.C.: Government Printing Office, 1970.

Texas. Department of Health. *Biennial Report*, 1950–52; 1952–54; 1954–56; 1956–58; 1958–60; 1960–62; 1962–64; 1964–66; 1966–68; 1968–70; 1970–72; 1972–74.

———— Department of Health Resources. *Biennial Report*, 1975–77.

———— Department of Public Welfare. *Annual Report*, 1947–69; 1971–73; 1975; 1976.

———— Department of Welfare. Blue Ribbon Task Force for the Evaluation of Medicaid, *Final Report: Recommendations and Issues*, 30 March 1977. Physicians' Subcommittee, *Provider Testimony*, 31 January 1977. Special Medical Services Subcommittee, *Expert Legislative and Staff Testimony*, 15 February 1977.

U.S. Comptroller General. *Attainable Benefits of the Medicaid Management Information System are Not Being Realized*. HRD 78-151. Washington, D.C.: General Accounting Office, 1978.

———— *Improved Administration Could Reduce the Costs of Ohio's Medicaid Program*. HRD-78-98. Washington, D.C.: General Accounting Office, 1978.

———— *The Swine Flu Program: An Unprecedented Venture into Preventive Medicine*. HRD 77-115. Washington, D.C.: General Accounting Office, 1977.

U.S. Congress. *Conference Report to Accompany H.R. 1, Social Security Amendments of 1972*. Rep. 1605. 92n Cong., 2d sess., 1972.

U.S. Congress. House. *Child Health Assessment Act: Hearings Before the Subcommittee on Health and the Environment of the Committee on Interstate and Foreign Commerce*. Serial No. 95-43. 95th Cong., 1st sess., 8–9 August 1977. [The date given in the title is incorrect; the hearings were held on 8–9 September 1977.]

———— Committee on Interstate and Foreign Commerce. *Child Health Assurance Act of 1978*. H. Rep. 95-1481 to Accompany H.R. 13611. 95th Cong., 2d sess., 1978.

———— Committee on Ways and Means. *Presidential Proposals for Revision in Social Security System: Hearings before the Committee on Ways and Means on H.R. 5710*. 90th Cong., 1st sess., 1–3 March 1967.

———— Committee on Ways and Means. *Section by Section Analysis and Explanation of Provisions of H.R. 5710, as Introduced on February 20, 1967*. 90th Cong., 1st sess., 1967.

———— *Report from the Committee on Interstate and Foreign Commerce to Accompany H.R. 10541*. 87th Cong., 2d sess., 18 June 1962.

———— *Social Security Amendments of 1967: Report of the Committee on Ways and Means on H.R. 12080*. H. Rep. 544. 90th Cong., 1st sess., 1967.

———— Subcommittee on Health and the Environment of the Committee on Interstate and Foreign Commerce. *A Discursive Dictionary of Health Care.* 94th Cong., 2d sess., February 1976.

———— Subcommittee on Health and the Environment of the Committee on Interstate and Foreign Commerce. *Data on the Medicaid Program: Eligibility, Services, Expenditures, Fiscal Years 1966–1977.* Washington, D.C.: Government Printing Office, 1977.

———— Subcommittee on Oversight and Investigation of the Committee on Interstate and Foreign Commerce. *Report: Department of Health, Education, and Welfare's Administration of Health Programs: Shortchanging Children.* 94th Cong., 2d sess., September 1976.

U.S. Congress. Senate. Committee on Government Operations. Subcommittee on Executive Reorganization and Government Research. *Report: Federal Role in Health.* 91st Cong., 2d sess., 30 April 1970.

———— Finance Committee. *Report to Accompany H.R. 1, Social Security Amendments of 1972.* S. Rep. 1230. 92d Cong., 2d sess., 1972.

———— *Social Security Amendments of 1967: Hearings before the Committee on Finance, United States Senate, on H.R. 12080.* 90th Cong., 1st sess., August 1967.

———— *Social Security Amendments of 1970: Report of the Committee on Finance, United States Senate, to Accompany H.R. 17550.* 91st Cong., 2d sess., 11 December 1970.

———— *Social Security Amendments of 1972: Conference Report to Accompany H.R. 1.* S. Rep. 92–1605. 92d Cong., 2d sess., 1972.

U.S. Department of Health, Education, and Welfare. "Ambulatory Medical Care Rendered in Pediatricians' Offices, 1975." National Center for Health Statistics. Advance Data No. 12, 13 October 1977.

———— *Child Health in America.* Pub. HSA 5015. Washington, D.C.: Government Printing Office, 1976.

———— *Children Who Received Physician's Services Under the Crippled Children's Program, 1955.* Maternal and Child Health Services Statistical Series No. 3, 1955.

———— *Children Who Received Physician's Services Under the Crippled Children's Program, 1970.* Maternal and Child Health Services Statistical Series No. 3, 1970.

———— *Children Who Received Physician's Services Under the Crippled Children's Program, 1971.* Maternal and Child Health Services Statistical Series No. 3, 1971.

———— *Data on the Medicaid Program: Eligibility, Services, Expenditures: Fiscal Years 1966–77.* Health Care Financing Administration. Institute for Medicaid Management, 1977.

———— *Data on the Medicaid Program: Eligibility/Services/Expenditures.* 1979 revised ed. Health Care Financing Administration. Medicare/Medicaid Institute, 1979.

———— *Graphic Presentation of Public Assistance and Related Data.* NCSS (National Center for Social Statistics) Report A-4, 1971.

———— *Handbook of Public Assistance Administration,* n.d.

———— *Health: United States, 1978.* Pub. No. 78–1232. December 1978.

———— *Immunizations Survey,* for the years 1967–1977.

———— *Maternal and Child Health Services in 1955.* Children's Bureau Statistical Series No. 38, 1957.

———— *Maternal and Child Health Services of State and Local Health Departments, Fiscal Year 1970.* Maternal and Child Health Statistical Series No. 2, 1971.

————— *Maternal and Child Health Services of State and Local Health Departments, Fiscal Years 1974, 1975, 1976.* Maternal and Child Health Statistical Series No. 13, 1979.

————— *Medicaid and Other Medical Care Financed from Public Assistance Funds*, FY 71. NCSS Report B-5, November 1972.

————— *Medicaid Children: Who Are They?* Social and Rehabilitation Service, 30 June 1971.

————— *Medicaid FY 1978–1982: Major Program Issues.* Social and Rehabilitation Service, September 1976.

————— *Medicaid Management Reports, Annual Report, Fiscal Year 1976.* Medical Services Administration, 1977.

————— *Medicaid Statistics, Fiscal Year 1976.* NCSS Report B-5, 1976.

————— *Numbers of Recipients and Amounts of Payments Under Medicaid, 1968.* NCSS, Report B-4, n.d.

————— *Numbers of Recipients and Amounts of Payments Under Medicaid, 1970.* NCSS Report B-4, 1972.

————— *Public Assistance Statistics.* NCSS Report A-2, May 1973.

————— *Understanding Medicaid: An Introduction to the Medical Services Administration*, 15 May 1975.

————— *Vendor Payments for Medical Care Under Public Assistance, Fiscal Years 1951–1970.* NCSS Report B-7, 6 July 1971.

————— Office of Child Health Affairs. *A Proposal for New Federal Leadership in Child and Maternal Health Care in the United States*, 23 February 1977.

U.S. Department of Labor. *Services for Crippled Children Under the Social Security Act: Development of Program, 1936–39.* Children's Bureau Publication No. 258, 1941.

Wholey, Joseph S., and Silver, George A. *Program Analysis: Maternal and Child Health Care Programs.* Washington, D.C.: Department of Health, Education, and Welfare, 1966.

EPSDT Program

Books and Articles

American Academy of Pediatrics. *Increased Professional Participation in State and Local EPSDT Programs.* Evanston, Ill.: American Academy of Pediatrics, 1976.

American Management Systems. *An Evaluative Study of Early and Periodic Screening, Diagnosis, and Treatment Program in Ohio and Wisconsin.* Arlington, Va.: American Management Systems, 1974.

American Orthopsychiatric Association. "Developmental Assessment in EPSDT." *American Journal of Orthopsychiatry* 48 (January 1978): 7–21.

Applied Management Sciences. *Assessment of EPSDT Practices and Costs.* Silver Springs, Md.: Applied Management Sciences, 1976.

Bokonon Systems, Inc. *EPSDT Status: A Review of 8 States.* Washington, D.C.: Bokonon Systems, Inc., 1974.

Boone Young & Associates. *Revised Interim Report on Evaluation of Head Start/EPSDT Collaborative Effort.* New York: Boone Young & Associates, 1976.

Bradley, Lindsey, Jr. "A Study of Broken Appointments for Pediatric Screening Examinations." Master's thesis, Trinity University, San Antonio, Texas, 1975.

Britt, Arthur E., and Dickson, Harold D. *Review of Shows for Treatment: EPSDT A Nine State Survey*. San Antonio: University of Texas Health Services Research Institute, 1977.

Children's Defense Fund. *EPSDT: Does it Spell Health Care for Poor Children?* Washington, D.C.: Children's Defense Fund, 1977.

Community Health Foundation. *Basic Issues in the Development of the Connecticut EPSDT Program*. Evanston, Ill.: Community Health Foundation, 1977.

——— *A Study of Broken Appointments in the Pennsylvania EPSDT Program*. Evanston, Ill.: Community Health Foundation, 1976.

Currier, Richard, "EPSDT: An Experience in Preventive Health." *Urban Health* 7 (April 1978):18–60.

——— "Michigan Leads in Screening Medicaid-eligible Children." *Michigan Medicine* 76 (March 1977):136–37.

Dickson, Harold D.; Evans, Harvey A.; Fiedler, Fred P.; Ellis, Carol; Pope, Janice; and Shippy, Ernest M. *EPSDT Diagnosis and Treatment Costs: A Five-State Analysis*. San Antonio: University of Texas Health Services Research Institute, 1978.

Dickson, Harold D.; Martin, Harry W.; and Davis, Sally. *Child Health in a Tri-Ethnic Rural Area—An EPSDT Demonstration in the Checkerboard Area of New Mexico*. San Antonio: University of Texas Health Services Institute, 1978.

Dykstra, Avis J. "Michigan's Experience in the Early and Periodic Screening, Diagnosis, and Treatment Program." *American Nurses' Association Publications* NP 47 (April 1975):43–49.

Fiedler, Fred. *Barrio Comprehensive Child Health Care Center—Final Report*. San Antonio: University of Texas Health Services Research Institute, 1975.

Foltz, Anne-Marie. "The Development of Ambiguous Federal Policy: Early and Periodic Screening, Diagnosis and Treatment (EPSDT)." *Milbank Memorial Fund Quarterly/Health and Society* 53 (Winter 1975):35–64.

——— *EPSDT: Lessons for National Health Insurance for Children*. Springfield, Va.: National Technical Information Service, 1975.

——— "The Impact of Federal Child Health Policy Under EPSDT: The Case of Connecticut." Yale Health Policy Project, Report No. 3. Yale University Department of Epidemiology and Public Health, New Haven, Ct., 1974.

——— "The Politics of Prevention: Child Health under Medicaid." Ph.D. Dissertation, Yale University, 1980.

Foltz, Anne-Marie, and Brown, Donna. "State Response to Federal Policy: Children, EPSDT, and the Medicaid Muddle." Medical Care 13 (August 1975): 630–642.

Gilliard, M. Elaine. *Medicaid for the Young: The Early and Periodic Screening, Diagnosis and Treatment Program in the South*. Atlanta, Ga: Southern Regional Council, 1976.

Greenberg, George D. "Federal Program Implementation in Selected States: A Study of the Implementation of the Partnership for Health Act and the Early and Periodic Screening, Diagnosis, and Treatment Program in Michigan, Pennsylvania, and Alabama." Report, Department of Political Science, University of Michigan, June 1979.

Health Services Research Institute. *EPSDT Demonstration in an Urban Setting, Dallas, Texas*. Final Evaluation Report, Phase 4: February 1976–June 1978. San Antonio: University of Texas Health Services Research Institute, 1978.

Kirk, Thomas R.; Rice, R. Gerald; and Allen, Paul M. "EPSDT—One Quarter Million Screenings in Michigan." *American Journal of Public Health* 66 (May 1976): 482–84.

Martin, Harry W., and Dickson, Harold D. *EPSDT Demonstration Projects: An Interim Evaluation, April 1974–March 1975.* San Antonio: University of Texas Health Services Research Institute, 1976.

Martin, Harry W.; Dickson, Harold D.; *et al. Impact of EPSTD—Summary. Phase II.* San Antonio: University of Texas Health Services Research Institute, 1972.

Peterson, Eric. *Legal Challenges to Bureaucratic Discretion: The Influence of Lawsuits on the Implementation of EPSDT.* PB 271 040. Springfield, Va.: National Technical Information Service, 1977.

Reis, Janet; Hughes, Edward F. X.; Pliska, S.; McCain, M. S.; Cordray, D.; Held, P.; Prince, T.; and Kerr, P. *An Assessment of the Validity of the Results of HCFA's Demonstration and Evaluation Programs for the Early and Periodic Screening, Diagnosis, and Treatment Program (EPSDT): A Metaevaluation.* Evanston, Ill.: Northwestern Center for Health Policy Studies, 1980.

Stimson, Wayne. *Demonstration in Follow-up: EPSDT Pierce County, Washington: Final Evaluation Report.* San Antonio: University of Texas Health Services Institute, 1979.

Government Documents

Frankenburg, William K., and North, A. Frederick. *A Guide to Screening for the Early and Periodic Screening, Diagnosis and Treatment Program under Medicaid.* Washington, D.C.: U.S. Department of Health, Education, and Welfare, 1974.

Michigan Departments of Social Services and Public Health. *EPSDT: Is Early Periodic Screening, Diagnosis and Treatment Achieving its Goal?* Report Period, January-June 1976.

Minnesota Senate Health Committee. *Minnesota's Progress in the EPSDT Program Development,* 21 February 1975.

U.S. Comptroller General. *Report to the Congress: Improvements Needed to Speed Implementation of Medicaid's Early and Periodic Screening, Diagnosis, and Treatment Program.* Washington, D.C.: General Accounting Office, 1975.

U.S. Department of Health, Education, and Welfare. "Comparison of EPSDT Program Costs for Present and Mandated Periodicity Schedules." Office of Child Health, Health Care Financing Administration, 7 December 1978.

———— *Field Staff Information and Instruction Series #158: Summary of EPSDT Progress Report for Period Ending March 31, 1973.* Social and Rehabilitation Service, Medical Services Administration, 8 June 1973.

———— *Field Staff Instruction and Information (FSII) Series, FY 74-16.* Social and Rehabilitation Service, Medical Services Administration, 1974.

———— *Medicaid: Early and Periodic Screening Diagnosis and Treatment for Individuals under 21.* PRG-21. Social and Rehabilitation Service, Medical Services Administration, 28 June 1972.

———— *Selected Characteristics of States' EPSDT Programs.* EPSDT Division, Social and Rehabilitation Service, Medical Services Administration, revised April 1977.

———— *Summary of Status Reports on Early and Periodic Screening and Diagnosis of Treatment.* Social and Rehabilitation Service, Medical Services Administration, September 1972.

Pediatric and Public Health Text and Reference Books

American Academy of Pediatrics. Committee on School Health. *School Health: A Guide for Health Professionals.* Evanston, Ill.: American Academy of Pediatrics, 1977.

———— Committee on Fetus & Newborn. *Standards and Recommendations for Hospital Care of Newborn Infants.* Evanston, Ill.: American Academy of Pediatrics, 1964.

———— Committee on Standards of Child Health Care. *Standards of Child Health Care.* 2d ed. Evanston, Ill.: American Academy of Pediatrics, 1972.

———— Committee on Standards of Child Health Care. *Standards of Child Health Care.* 3d ed. Evanston, Ill.: American Academy of Pediatrics, 1977.

———— Council on Pediatric Practice. *Standards of Child Health Care.* Evanston, Ill.: American Academy of Pediatrics, 1967.

———— *Report of the Committee on Infectious Diseases* (Red Book). Evanston, Ill.: American Academy of Pediatrics, 1977.

Arena, Jay M., ed. *Davison's Compleat Pediatrician.* 9th ed. Philadelphia: Lea and Febiger, 1969.

Barness, Lewis A. *Manual of Pediatric Physical Diagnosis.* 4th ed. Chicago: Year Book Medical Publishers, 1972.

Barnett, Henry L., with collaboration of Einhorn, Arnold H., eds. *Pediatrics.* 14th ed. New York: Appleton-Century-Crofts, 1968.

Barnett, Henry L., and Einhorn, Arnold H., eds. *Pediatrics.* 15th ed. New York: Appleton-Century-Crofts, 1972.

Bass, Lee W., and Wolfson, Jerome H. *The Style and Management of Pediatric Practice.* Pittsburgh: University of Pittsburgh Press, 1977.

Clark, Duncan W., and MacMahon, Brian, eds. *Preventive Medicine.* Boston: Little, Brown, 1967.

Davison, Wilburt C. *The Compleat Pediatrician.* Durham, N.C.: Duke University Press, 1934.

Davison, Wilburt C., and Levinthal, Jeana Davison. *The Compleat Pediatrician: Practical, Diagnostic, Therapeutic, and Preventive Pediatrics.* 8th ed. Durham, N.C.: Duke University Press, 1961.

Forfar, John O., and Arneil, Gavin C., eds. *Textbook of Paediatrics.* Edinburgh and London: Churchill Livingstone, 1973.

Gellis, Sydney Paul, and Kagan, Benjamin M. *Current Pediatric Therapy 3.* 3d ed. Philadelphia: W. B. Saunders, 1968.

———— *Current Pediatric Therapy 8.* 8th ed. Philadelphia: W. B. Saunders, 1978.

Green, Morris, and Haggerty, Robert, eds. *Ambulatory Pediatrics.* Philadelphia: W. B. Saunders, 1968.

———— *Ambulatory Pediatrics II.* 2d ed. Philadelphia: W. B. Saunders, 1977.

Green, Morris, and Richmond, Julius. *Pediatric Diagnosis: Interpretation of Signs and Symptoms in Different Age Periods.* Philadelphia: W. B. Saunders, 1954.

———— *Pediatric Diagnosis: Interpretation of Signs and Symptoms in Different Age Periods.* 2d ed. Philadelphia: W. B. Saunders, 1962.

Hanlon, John J. *Principles of Public Health Administration.* St. Louis: C. V. Mosby, 1964.

Harper, Paul A. *Preventive Pediatrics: Child Health and Development*. New York: Appleton-Century-Crofts, 1962.

Hilleboe, Herman E., and Larimore, Granville W., eds. *Preventive Medicine*. Philadelphia: W. B. Saunders, 1959.

―――― *Preventive Medicine*. 2d ed. Philadelphia: W. B. Saunders, 1965.

Holt, L. Emmet. *Diseases of Infancy and Childhood*. New York: Appleton, 1897.

Holt, L. Emmet, Jr., and McIntosh, Rustin, eds. *Holt's Diseases of Infancy and Childhood*. 10th ed. New York: Appleton, 1933.

―――― *Holt's Pediatrics*. 12th ed. New York: Appleton-Century-Crofts, 1953.

Holt, L. Emmet, Jr.; McIntosh, Rustin; and Barnett, Henry L. *Pediatrics*. 13th ed. New York: Appleton-Century-Crofts, 1962.

Hull, David, ed. *Recent Advances in Paediatrics*. 5th ed. Edinburgh: Churchill Livingstone, 1976.

Illingworth, Ronald S. *The Development of the Infant and Young Child: Normal and Abnormal*. 6th ed. London: Churchill Livingstone, 1975.

―――― *The Normal Child: Some Problems of the Early Years and their Treatment*. 6th ed. London: Churchill Livingstone, 1975.

Leavell, Hugh Rodman, and Clark, E. Gurney. *Textbook of Preventive Medicine*. New York: McGraw-Hill, 1953.

――――, eds. *Textbook of Preventive Medicine*. 3d ed. New York: McGraw-Hill, 1965.

McKendry, J.B.J., and Bailey, J. D. *The Infant and Pre-Schooler: Pediatric Problems in Family Practice*. Don Mills: Longman Canada, 1974.

Nelson, Waldo E., ed. *Textbook of Pediatrics*. 5th ed. Philadelphia: W. B. Saunders, 1950.

Oberst, Byron B. *Practical Guidance for Office Pediatric and Adolescent Practice*. Springfield, Ill.: Charles C. Thomas, 1973.

Rendle-Short, John. *The Child: A Guide for the Paediatric Team*. 2d ed. Bristol: John Wright, 1977.

Rudolph, Abraham M., ed. *Pediatrics*. 16th ed. New York: Appleton-Century-Crofts, 1977.

Sartwell, Philip E., ed. *Preventive Medicine and Public Health*. New York: Appleton-Century-Crofts, 1973.

Shirkey, Harry C., ed. *Pediatric Therapy*. 5th ed. St. Louis: C. V. Mosby, 1975.

Silver, Henry K.; Kempe, C. Henry; and Bruyn, Henry B. *Handbook of Pediatrics*. Los Altos, Calif.: Lange Medical Publications, 1955.

―――― *Handbook of Pediatrics*. 12th ed. Los Altos, Calif.: Lange Medical Publications, 1977.

Smith, David W., ed. *Introduction to Clinical Pediatrics*. 2d ed. Philadelphia: W. B. Saunders, 1977.

Thompson, Hugh C., and Seagle, Joseph B. *The Management of Pediatric Practice: A Philosophy and Guide*. Springfield, Ill.: Charles C. Thomas, 1961.

Vaughan, Victor C. III, and McKay, R. James, eds. *Nelson Textbook of Pediatrics*. 10th ed. Philadelphia: W. B. Saunders, 1975.

Wasserman, Edward, and Slobody, Lawrence B. *Survey of Clinical Pediatrics*. 6th ed. New York: McGraw-Hill, 1974.

West, Kelly M.; Wender, Ruth W.; and May, Ruby S. "Books in Clinical Practice 1971–1975." *Postgraduate Medicine* 56 (December 1974): 60–81.

Ziai, Mohsen, ed. *Pediatrics*. 2d ed. Boston: Little, Brown, 1975.

Index

Abbot, Grace, 131
Aesculapius, 121–24, 164
Aid to families with dependent
  children
  and penalty regulations, 36, 66–67 (see
  also Penalty regulations)
  Texas Welfare Dept., 85–86
Allison, Graham T., 5
Altman, Lawrence K., 226 n. 124
Amend, Wesley, 213 n. 168
American Academy of Orthopedic Sur-
  geons, 25
American Academy of Pediatrics, 9,
  113, 137
  and child health standards, 132–35
  and infant mortality, 125
  screening criticized by, 68
  and well-child examinations, 149–54.
  See also Pediatricians; Physicians
American Association for Psychiatric
  Services for Children, 148
American Cerebral Palsy Association,
  25
American Medical Association
  periodic exams promoted by, 122
  public health defined by, 89
American Nursing Association, 26
American Orthopsychiatric Associa-
  tion, 148
American Parents' Committee, 25–26
American Pediatric Society, 137. See also
  American Academy of Pediatrics;
  Pediatricians
American Public Health Association,
  88–89, 138
  Control of Communicable Disease in Man,
  141
American Public Welfare Association,
  80
Anemia, 130; 222 n. 62
Annual reports
  Connecticut Health Dept., 89–93
  Connecticut Welfare Dept., 80–83
  Texas Health Dept., 93–97
  Texas Welfare Dept., 83–88
Arizona, Medicaid nonparticipation by,

64; 207 n. 7
Association of Schools of Public Health,
  138
Association of State and Territorial
  Health Officers, 25

Baker, Josephine S., 223 n. 81
Bardach, Eugene, 8
Bureaucratic ideology. See Ideology
Bureaucratic relationships
  and health and welfare department ri-
  valry, 43
  and MSA-MCHS rivalry, 31
Burke, James A., 26

Califano, Joseph, 39–40, 69
California
  EPSDT program, 52
  methods of cutting costs, 56
Carter, President Jimmy, and CHAP,
  73–74
Case finding, 15, 26–28
  costs, 58
  methods, 47
Case management
  Connecticut, 103–7
  Texas, 110–13, 172
Center for Disease Control, 142
  and swine flu immunization, 155–57
Children, preventive medicine for,
  124–29
Children and Youth clinics, 15–16
  Seattle project, 133
Children's Bureau, 14–16
  child health responsibility of, 132–33
  demise of, 133–34
  Infant Care, 136 n. 79
  philosophy of service, 21. See also
  American Academy of Pediatrics;
  Pediatricians
Children's Defense Fund
  and CHAP, 72–74
  and developmental assessment, 148
  and follow-ups, 54–55
  and penalty reviews, 70; 208 n. 33
Chin, Dr. James, 226 n. 124

Closed systems, 3
  Texas screening as example of, 109,
    174
Cohen, Wilbur, 30
Committee on the Costs of Medical
  Care, 122
Communicable Disease Center. See
  Center for Disease Control
Community Health Foundation, 104
Compliance procedures, weakness of,
  64–65
Comprehensive care, 119; 216 n. 1
  Rochester experiment in, 129; 221 n.
    58
Comprehensive Employment Training
  Act, Connecticut staffing for, 104–5
Connecticut
  bureaucratic constraints in, 114
  case management in, 103–7
  EPSDT program established by, 101–2
  Health Dept., 89–93, 96–97, 171–72
  information systems, 102–3
  institutional constraints in, 115–16
  management system's effects in, 106–7
  periodicity schedules in, 161
  referral patterns in, 54–55
  Welfare Dept., 80–83, 87–88, 171
Connecticut Medical Society, 158
Consultative services
  Connecticut Health Dept., 92
  Texas Health Dept., 95–96
Cost
  of Medicaid/EPSDT services, 32–33,
    56–59
  of MMIS in Texas, 109
  of outreach workers in Texas, 112
  of Texas screening, 108–9
Courtney, Gavin S., 208 n. 30
Crippled Children's Program, 14–15,
    119
  case finding in, 15, 26–28
  children served by, 26; 200 n. 59
  and Connecticut Health Dept., 91
  and preventive care mandate, 24
  registries in, 14–16
  and Texas Health Dept., 96
Cuban missile crisis, 5

Davis, David W., 63
Davis, Karen, 72–73; 198 n. 28
Day care programs, 132
Decision-making. See Incrementalism

Definitions
  comprehensive care, 119; 216 n. 1
  health maintenance, 120
  ideology, 78
  politics, 8
  prevention, 7–8
  preventive medicine, 120
  primary care, 119–20
  public health, 89
  public welfare, 80
  screening, 44, 120
Delphi method, 137
Dental service, 54–55
  of Texas Health Dept., 95, 108; 215 n.
    196
Denver Developmental Screening Test,
  147–48
Derthick, Martha, 6, 172, 233
Developmental assessment, 145–146
  consensus on, 145–49, 153–54
  screening distinguished from, 146
  and testing, 147–48. See also Screening
Disease
  and children's preventive medicine
    needs, 126–27
  diphtheria, 127
  publications about, 141–42
  setting standards to prevent, 129–30.
    See also Immunization; Standards

Early and Periodic Screening, Diagnosis, and Treatment
  administering agency, 29–32
  costs and funding, 32–33, 56–59
  critics and advocates, 2, 53; 205 n. 131
  eligibility, 26–27, 33
  EPSDT amendment (1967), 24
  HEW's policy characterized, 37–42, 66
  legislative history, 25–29
  management tasks, 99
  origins, 1, 13, 22–29
  requirements, 1
  services, 33–35, 44–56
  state administration, 42–44
  states' view of, 59
  success, 2, 167
  why it went awry, 168–77. See also Eli-
    gibility; Penalty regulations; Case
    management
Elementary and Secondary Education
  Act, implementation study of, 5–6
Eligibility
  EPSDT, 26–27, 33

Medicaid, 19
regulations, 41–42. *See also* Means test
Eliot, Martha M., 26
Emergency Maternity and Infant Care
  program
  Children's Bureau's implementation,
  133, 136
  enactment, 21
ERO v. Mahler, 214 n. 187
Evaluation research, 4; 195 n. 10

Family, child health responsibility of,
  131–32
Family Health Insurance Plan, 32
Farm Security Agency, 126
Fawcett, Thomas M., 208 n. 28
Federalism and federal-state relations,
  63, 115–16, 173
Fogarty International Center, 138
Follow-ups of screening
  costs, 58
  Tracer Evaluation Project, 51; 205 n.
  130
  variations in state patterns, 53–55
Ford, President Gerald R., and swine
  flu immunization, 155–57
Foundation for the Blind, 25
Fuoroli, Alfred G., 214 n. 188

Galdston, Iago, 218 n. 13
Gates, Dr. Philip A., 108
Grants, compliance procedures and,
  64–65
Grasso, Governor Ella, 71; 208 n. 36

Hargrove, Erwin C., 195 n. 10
Harris, Robert, 228 n. 159
Harris v. Davis, 205 n. 128
Hart, J. T., 218 n. 12
Health care providers
  Connecticut, 102, 107
  cost problems, 57
  finding, 45–47, 174
Health departments
  and state Medicaid administration,
  42–44. *See also* Public health; Title V;
  Ideology
Health, Education and Welfare Dept.
  Program Analysis, 22, 169, 177
  responsibilities under EPSDT, 38–39
  vacillating policy of, 37–41, 66
Health maintenance, 120
  Kaiser-Permanente Group

Health Plan, 123, 147, 153
Health systems, 3
Holland, W. W., 120, 123
Holt, L. Emmet, 225 n. 103
Hygeia, 121–24, 164

Ideology, 78
  Connecticut Health Dept., 89–93, 96–
  97, 175
  Connecticut Welfare Dept., 80–83, 87–
  88, 101, 172, 174–75
  EPSDT implementation, 97–98, 172
  and goals, 78–79
  Texas Health Dept., 93–97, 172, 175
  Texas Welfare Dept., 83–88, 172, 174–
  75
Illinois Commission on Children, 25
Immunization
  consensus on, 139–45, 153–54
  discrepancies in standards and practice of, 143–45
  mandates for, 140–41
  of nonwhite children, 145
  policy's purpose, 142
  "Red Book" recommendations, 144
  for rubella in Connecticut, 157–59
  for smallpox, 139–40
  states mandating, 141
  swine flu program of, 155–57. *See also*
  Disease
Implementation research, 4–6; 195 n.
  10
Incrementalism
  decision-making illustrated, 4–5, 13,
  59–60
  and why EPSDT went awry, 175–77
Indiana
  EPSDT program, 52
  noncompliance with Public Assis
  tance, 65
Infant mortality rates, 125
Institutions
  constrainsts on policy, 6–7, 63–116,
  171–175
  intellectual traditions in, 4–6. *See also*
  Ideology
Iron deficiency anemia, 130; 222 n. 62

Johnson, President Lyndon
  child health initiatives, 1, 22–23
  Great Society programs, bibliography,
  195 n. 9
Johnston, Marlin, 211 n. 108, 216 n. 222

Joint Committee on Mental Health of Children, 137, 146

Kaiser-Permanente Group Health Plan, 123, 147, 153
Kemler, Joan, 214 n. 187
Kessner, David, 130

Lesser, Dr. Arthur, 30
Lewis, John, 228 n. 158
Lindblom, Charles, 5; 196 nn. 12, 15
Lustick, Ian, 176

Magnuson, Senator Warren, 133
Martz, Samuel, 207 nn. 11, 12
Maternal and Child Health Programs, 15–16
    MSA rivalry, 31
    Texas Health Dept., 95–96. See also Title V
Maternity and infant care projects, 15–16
    Connecticut Health Dept., 91
Matthews, F. David, 69
McCarthy, Brian, 214 n. 179
McIntosh, Harold, 104–5
Means test
    Avoidance in EMIC program, 21
    Medicaid and Title V contrasted, 21–22
    Public Health Service, 21
    public programs without, 133; 222 n. 70. See also Eligibility
Meany, George, 25
Medicaid
    administration by states, 42–44
    children served, 26; 200 n. 59
    Connecticut Welfare Dept., 80
    costs, 56–59
    criticisms, 100
    decentralization, 40, 70, 75
    eligibility, 19
    financing and services, 20
    origins and provisions, 16–18
    staffing, 38–39
    Texas, 86, 107, 109
    Title V contrasted, 20–22
Medical Management Information Systems, 43–44, 99–101
    Connecticut, 102–3
    Texas, 109–10
Medical Services Administration
    EPSDT administrator, 30–31
    MCHS rivalry, 31

Mental health and developmental assessment, 146–47
Michigan, EPSDT implementation by, 47, 52; 204 n. 125
Miller, C. Arden, 132
Mills, Wilbur, and EPSDT amendment, 23–24
Moore, Beatrice, 39
Morgan, Chester W., 228 n. 160
Morrell, Joyce, 205 n. 128
Morrison, James, 198 n. 17
Multiphasic health checkup, 123, 153; 218 n. 21

National Association of Counties, 71
National Education Association, school health appraisals by, 138
National Governors' Conference, 71
National Health Council periodic exams, 122
National health insurance, EPSDT as lesson for, 178–79
National Institutes of Health, consensus conferences by, 169–70
National Journal, 38
National Legal Program on Health Problems of the Poor, 34
Neuhauser, Duncan, 164
New Haven Register, 157
New towns in-town program, 6, 172
New York Academy of Medicine, 129
Nursing
    and Connecticut Health Dept., 91–92
    and Texas EPSDT, 108
Nutrition, Children's Bureau's standards for, 136

Oakland Project, 6, 169
Open system, 3
    Connecticut as example of, 174, 175
Organizational ideology. See Ideology

Pediatricians
    as child advocates, 138
    and sources of competition, 133–35
    and standards for child care, 132–33, 136–38, 163–64. See also American Academy of Pediatrics
Penalty regulations
    and AFDC funds, 36, 66–67
    federalism's limiting effects on, 75–77
    history of, 65–67

noncomplying states, 66–67
reasons for failure of, 67–76
vacillating policy's effect on, 37
Periodic health examinations
frequency of visits, 149–53
multiple screening as form of, 123
origins, 121–24, 128
validity of, 139
Periodicity schedules
Connecticut, 162
state practices, 159–62
states' problems, 45
Texas, 162
Phenylketonuria (PKU), 127, 136
Physicians
Medicaid participation by, 45–46, 102, 175
pediatricians' conflict with, 135
periodic exams importance for, 122; 218 n. 13
Texas, 93–94. See also Health Care Providers; Pediatricians; Texas Medical Association
Polaris missile program, 99
implementation study of, 6, 7
Poliomyelitis vaccines, 140
Poliomyelitis Vaccine Assistance Act, 142
Politics, 8
Powers, Galen, 207 n. 13, 208 n. 34
Press, Stephen, 104–5
Pressman, Jeffrey L., and Oakland Project, 6, 169, 237
Prevention, 7–8
Preventive care, 15
and Crippled Children's program, 24, 29
setting standards for, 129–30
Preventive medicine 7–8, 120
and children's special needs, 124–29
Primary care, 119–20
Professional Standards Review Organizations, 136
Public health, 88–89
Connecticut, 89–93, 96–97
Texas, 93–97
Public Health Service, and Children's Bureau's demise, 133–34
Public welfare, 80
Connecticut, 80–83, 87–88
Texas, 83–88
Pure milk movement, 128

Record keeping, states' difficulties with, 43–44
"Red Book," 142–45; 224 n. 90
Referrals. See Follow-ups
Regulations
Connecticut Health Dept., 92
eligibility qualifications, 41–42 (see also Eligibility)
EPSDT, 29–35. See also Penalty regulations
Reimbursement, interagency rivalry over, 30–31. See also Bureaucratic relationships
Research, 4; 195 n. 10
Ribicoff, Senator Abraham, 18, 32, 36, 70
Rogers, Paul, 40
Rubella, 157–59, 170
Ryan, William F., 36

Sackett, David L., 123
Sanford, Terry, 63
Sapolsky, Harvey, and Polaris missile study, 6, 7, 99
Schools
child health care programs in, 134–35
NEA's health appraisals of, 138
Screening, 44, 120
cervical cancer conference, 170; 228 n. 2
for children's diseases, 127–28
children eligible for, 41–42
of Connecticut children, 107
consensus lacking on, 7, 53–54, 163–165, 168–71 (see also Developmental assessment; well-child examination)
costs estimated, 22–23
developmental (see Developmental assessment)
efficiency of, 139; 224 n. 98
expenditures for, 53
frequency under EPSDT, 169–163
HEW Program Analysis and, 159, 177
penalties for failure to implement, 36 (see also Penalty regulations)
and periodic health exams compared, 122
for Phenylketonuria (PKU), 127, 136
procedures recommended, 44–45, 159; 228 n. 163
purpose and types of, 14–15
recommended visits, table of, 150, 152
reporting problems, 47–48

Screening (cont.)
  state practice, 159–62
  Texas, 108–13
Seattle Children and Youth Project, 133
Shapiro, Bernard, 80, 82
Sheppard-Towner Act, 13–14, 125
Silver, George A., 199 n. 40
Smallpox immunization, 139–140
Smith, Dr. Donald C., 28
Social Security Act
  Immunity from political tinkering, 176
  Title V (see Title V)
  Title XIX (see Medicaid)
South Carolina, EPSDT program in, 52
Staffing
  Connecticut Welfare Dept., 82, 103–6
  shortages, 38–39
  state Medicaid departments, 43
  Texas Welfare Dept., 84
Standards
  child health responsibility, 131–35
  pediatricians' role, 136–38, 163–64
  PSROs, 136
  purpose of setting, 129–30. See also
    American Academy of Pediatrics;
    Pediatricians
Standards of Child Health Care, 145, 151
Steiner, Gilbert Y., 66
Stickler, Gunnar B., 227 n. 152
Stuart, Bruce, 198 n. 26
Sundquist, James L., 63
Swine flu immunization program, 155–
  57, 170

Testing in developmental assessment,
  147–48
Texas
  bureaucratic constraints, 114
  case management and effects, 110–13
  developmental assessment, 147–48
  EPSDT program, 52, 55, 107–113
  Health Dept., 93–97, 171–72
  institutional constraints, 115–16
  MMIS, 109–10
  periodicity schedules, 162
  Welfare Dept., 83–88, 171
Texas Medical Association, 93, 113, 172,
  175
Title V
  history, 13–16
  Medicaid contrasted, 20–22
  screening services, 46
  services described, 14–16. See also

Health departments; Medicaid; Public health
Tracer Evaluation Project, 205 n. 130
Transportation in Texas EPSDT, 108,
  111

Umbrella agencies, state medicaid administration of, 42–44
Understanding Medicaid, 38

Vaccination. See Immunization
Vaccine Assistance Act, 142

"War on Cancer," 171
Weatherhogg, C. R., 208 n. 26
Webb, Jr., Dr. Charles R., 226 n. 124
Weikel, Keith, 208 n. 30, 202 n. 89
Weinberger, Caspar, 39
Welfare. See Public welfare
Welfare agencies, as state Medicaid ad-
  ministrators, 42–44. See also Ideology
Well-child conference, 15, 128. See also
  Periodic health examinations; Well-
  child examinations
Well-child examinations
  consensus on, 149–54
  discrepancies in standards for, 153
  frequency of visits, 149–53
Wessel, Morris A., 214 n. 183
Wholey, Joseph S., 199 n. 37
Wildavsky, Aaron B., and Oakland Pro-
  ject, 6, 169, 237
Winslow, C. E. A., 11
Woods, Marion, 208 n. 27
Wyoming, screening in, 48, 50

Yankauer, Alfred, 151